AF342703

The Rise and Fall of Health Care in America

Ted Nolan Thompson, M.D.

AF342703

SAVANT INFORMATION PUBLISHING

Copyright Feb. 26, 2003
by Ted Nolan Thompson, M.D.

All rights reserved. No part of this non dramatic literary work may be reproduced or transmitted in any form or by any means, electronic or mechanical, including photocopying, recording or by information storage and retrieval system without written permission of the author except where permitted by law.

Library of Congress Cataloging in publication data: Copyright No. TXu 1 - 082 - 138
Ted Nolan Thompson, M.D.

To The Memory of

FRANCIS SCOTT SMYTH, MD
Professor of Pediatrics

DEAN
The School of Medicine
University of California
San Francisco
U.S.A.
The Nineteen Fifties

AS OF 2005 ALL ATTEMPTS FOR REFORM
HAVE FAILED

BUT

THERE IS NO STATUTE OF LIMITATION
ON SINS THAT CRY OUT TO HEAVEN

TABLE OF CONTENTS

INTRODUCTION

During the tragic period of World War II there occurred a giant leap in medical care by virtue of the introduction of both sulfa and penicillin. In addition, while war cannot be a better way to advance care of the ill and injured, there did occur an improved understanding involving the management of numerous kinds of war related traumas particularly burns and those relating to peripheral nerves.

Following World War II there has been a trend determined to make the practice of medicine totally scientific. Regardless after fifty years, specifically as of the year 2003, and in spite of emphasis on sophisticated technology, medical care remains more "art" than "science."

Rather than come to the realization that knowledge acquired in molecular biology, biophysics and biochemistry, while tremendously helpful in "explaining disease," cannot readily be applied to curing the desperately ill, risks and uncertainties have been added to human suffering that have been either de-emphasized or hidden behind eagerness and hype.

While amazing strides have been made that relate for instance to correcting abnormal cardiac rhythms as well as abnormal heart valve function, the mystery of heart muscle has not been solved. While very impressive advances in the treatment of joint disease have alleviated terrible suffering, particularly through joint replacement, the treatment and understanding of rheumatoid arthritis has remained far short of the mark.

While it's true when something goes wrong with the nervous system it goes wrong in a certain way and this, by the way, can be determined with just "clinical" expertise, colossal disappointments remain for fully understanding Parkinson's disease first identified by James Parkinson in 1817! Multiple sclerosis is not yet fully understood. Its description as a separate disease dates back to Jean Martin Charcot at the Salpetriere in Paris France, and the year 1868!

Regardless of all new very sophisticated technological equipment, "backwardness" best exemplifies pharmacological treatment for control of the symptoms of the epilepsies during the past three decades. Across the board seizure symptom cases do not receive anywhere near as good or as considerate care as they received in the nineteen sixties. While underlying mechanisms may well be better understood such fails to benefit the patients! All a patient desires is to get rid of the tendency to have spells. The situation is similar regarding treatment and control of the many various forms of mental illness. The mentally ill patient simply wants medication(s) or some therapeutic procedure to feel better. The "why" of their illness is of academic interest to the psychiatrist, not necessarily the patient.

Public awareness of an insistence to over utilize expensive and sophisticated technological equipment, along with a general perception that half of all surgical procedures are unnecessary has opened the door understandably for various forms of alternative health care. A breakdown of the physician-patient relationship over the past 20 years furthered a desire for alternative treatment methods defined by many as dubiously helpful but at the least without any risk of being harmful. As a greater proportion of the population becomes more fearful of doctors and hospitals, an uninsured population has panicked over costs whenever some unexpected illness or injury occurs.

For treatment even the so-called "sugar pill" has value if administered with conviction. The reverse of this has repeatedly been shown when effects of powerful specifically targeted pharmaceutical products are tested in the "double blind" situation. Upon breaking the code a "placebo" has caused certain side-effects, as did the medication. The phenomenal ability of certain medicines to reach their target and perform "exactly" as intended have in all too many instances become a patient's undoing when these products are offered far beyond the "expertise and experience" of many physicians. A deficiency of medical center teaching in the fundamentals of pharmacology along with careless use of so many available pharmaceuticals in recent years has become another reason for alternative therapies, whether herbs from the health food store, acupuncture or chiropractic manipulation.

Where alternative medicine is concerned more scientifically oriented doctors are best cautious about criticism because, if there were no value to various therapies that do seem odd, why so much testimony to the contrary? Until the "secrets of the human body" are more fully explained in a scientific, predictable, reproducible way there will continue to be a seemingly unusual treatment for even very serious conditions with hearsay from intelligent people about a definite value.

Among the first documented deaths thought due to Chinese herbs, it was discovered in San Francisco California during the nineteen-fifties a Western medication was mixed with an herbal remedy. An example was the adding of phenylbutazone, a very effective pain medication. The phenylbutazone was capable of causing an unlikely side effect of suppressing certain essential blood elements produced in one's bone marrow. Lack of knowledge on the part of both the giver and the taker of the remedy led to a preventable death. Relying too enthusiastically upon "Internet information" has taken people down the "highway of undesirable results" An Internet example has been the recommendation of zinc chloride (ZnCl2), a poisonous antiseptic, disinfectant, mixed with pokeweed purple root for skin cancers. A more agreeable approach for the victim of "Internet self inflicted injury" was one designed by dermatologists and plastic surgeons to get rid of the disease producing cells, without eradicating normal skin as well as cartilage!

Due to burgeoning knowledge how to teach medical students to be the most helpful kinds of physicians within the classic four years period that prepares students for internship is a problem of major proportions! There's a gradual departure from teaching to be a "clinical diagnostician," to make sound medical judgments based on whether the patient generally "looks and acts healthy." Instruments such as the stethoscope, ophthalmoscope, otoscope, reflex hammer with an additional x-ray of the chest and electrocardiogram (EKG), are ignored. There's "a new breed of practicing molecular biologists," prone to excessive, expensive testing that threatens to replace altogether not just the stethoscope but also the all-important "medical history" as well as the "physical examination!" Based on what we "really know as of 2003" this trend becomes very counter productive and impractical, let alone extremely expensive!

As we entered the new century it's not difficult to trace the relative cost of some medical care back to the mid-sixties. Less than forty years ago one kind of hospitalized case cost just $250. The same cases today and the very same "effective medical treatment" have run as high as $30,000!

Medical care cost hovers at 14% of America's gross national product in spite of "managed care." (Canada's costs just 9% of their GNP). Overlooking sound economics too many physicians, and perhaps nearly all Ph.D. researchers, remain increasingly focused, or even obsessed, with a future era of gene therapies bordering on the impossible. Even if such were possible one logically envisages such notions as absolutely unaffordable to over 99% of American society!

Lack of confidence in American physicians along with public awareness of available high technology leads to increasing numbers of anxiously concerned to be "scanned." Indeed there's "endoscopy," "sonography," "radiography," "computed tomography," as well as "mammography" and non-x-ray "magnetic resonance imaging." For the latter a patient is positioned in a magnetic field chamber while radio wave signals are conducted. Their released energy is then computer programmed to formulate sharp imagery at the lipid (fat)–water interface." Over two decades nuclear medicine advances way beyond the old thyroid-uptake test to include a great variety of scans of heart, lung, liver and bone density (the DEXA scan) as well as the famous two photon or positron-emission-tomogram (the PET scan) that measures radioactive glucose uptake in the brain. While all such equipment and tests are fascinating and such achievements are very worthy of scientific praise such testing is widely over utilized for simply commercial reasons.

Radiologists, doctors set apart from actually managing patients, justify the usage of such tests as "reality testing" to allay patient's worries, when in truth it's first and foremost "part of wide spread commercialism in response to what the public wants." The trend overlooks the major truth the lay public is not in a position to actually know what is "strategically best." As "screening for findings" precedes the clinical awareness of disease poor judgment or lack of good judgment follows as surgeons with "eyes on business" rely too much on the radiologist. Such tactics for approaching disease not only begs a question whether it's sensible or necessary to go through four years of medical school, but also calls for an analogy: "if such military tactics were employed one could be certain the war would be lost!"

History teaches that with certain passages of time there is the expectancy of death. This can result from plagues, cancers, strokes, heart and vascular disease as well as other serious ills. In this modern age man deals with "fumes." Regardless an adequate population within civilization continues to survive and push on to hopefully progress to better things. Perhaps if we used our knowledge to best advantage surviving to the age of one hundred years would be commonplace. There is, however, very little confidence in that now, at least in terms of "quality years."

A major threat to probably all societies, society defined as the sum of interpersonal relationships among a given population, is the increasing number of mentally ill, whether from genetics, nurturing, brainwashing or drug abuse. As things stand mental illness (not AIDs) may most certainly be the most threatening problem facing America and the world today! In view of this it's terribly disappointing to learn that mental illness may be the least funded among disease programs!

As for the 21st century being the "century of the gene," it's worth noting it's been nearly 20 years since the single gene defect for cystic fibrosis (mucoviscidosis) was identified. It has not been possible to deliver that single corrective DNA sequence to the appropriate cells to correct this problem with present techniques (adenovirus vector). Sickle cell disease, likewise just a single gene mutation, hasn't been correctable either. Though the French have reported apparent success with such treatment directed against a form of immunodeficiency (Science 288,669,2000) and this provides some encouragement scientifically, if not economically, it is folly to discuss "cancer treatments" by means of such methods when conceivably the estimate of 25 to 50 genes are involved! Furthermore, as of 2002 encouragement turned to discouragement when the French transplant experiment caused a case of leukemia. The very cost alone of such therapeutic experiments and proposals has proven to be enough to stagger financial minds in terms of what can be reasonably allocated for illness among America's population even with complete success or no failures whatsoever.

When "DNA" is mentioned, remember, it's not just a simple matter of properly sequencing the four bases, namely: adenine, thymine, cytosine and guanine. Even the methylation of DNA poses a major problem because "it inactivates so-called promoter genes." Among many things suspected the very cause of cancer as well as pre-mature aging might well be, as stated, related to methylation of DNA!

As for the cloning of a normal human being stem cell research simply cannot lead to that! Any albeit unlikely result would be "an accelerated aged version of the person being cloned with defects both mentally and physically too numerous to mention!" Discussions about the morality and ethical issues over and above the economics of such procedures are undoubtedly of sociological interest, however, from a scientific viewpoint should, practically speaking, not even be entertained. One dare not be really serious to say otherwise.

TED NOLAN THOMPSON, MD
November 2005

CHAPTER I

"THE FREE ENTERPRISE SYSTEM AND HEALTH CARE IN AMERICA"

By1938, during the latter part of the Great Depression, fee for service delivery of medical care had had its' shortcomings for several years. It was well known physicians at times performed their services for no pay. Moreover physicians were willing to do so. Once in awhile it was a pleasure. Physician-sons' of physicians remembered their doctor-father staying all night at a patients' home. He administered morphine periodically until daybreak to help alleviate agony, with such appropriate medications and moral support, until at last the patient passed that kidney stone.

Soon after sun-up it was time for breakfast. Following handshakes, along with hugs and tears of gratitude, "Doc" went ahead and joined the family for several cups of coffee and some breakfast. It was understood from the very start there simply was no means whereby the physician would be paid in money. For all too many there was very little money. In those days a cup of coffee in an "FBI cup" cost a nickel. A loaf of bread was hardly more than ten cents. A good hair cut cost a quarter.

Doc left directly for his office. Having had just a few short naps he was a little surprised not having too much trouble staying awake for the day's patient load. That great feeling, you helped someone in need, kept you going for a while at least. Furthermore times were tough for so many. Arriving home 33 hours after being away was wonderful. No one complained. Only good things were said, but there were private thoughts before dad at last went to bed. No matter how you reasoned, it was thought better all around if the doctor could have skipped the breakfast and simply gotten paid.

Henry John Kaiser, American industrialist, thought exactly that; that physicians ought to get paid. In 1938 the energetic, colorful, very successful road, dam and bridge builder, soon to become a civilian hero of World War II, set up a prepaid medical care plan for his employees, the very first health maintenance organization (HMO), in Oakland, California. It was given a name: "Kaiser-Permanente."

After World War II membership in Kaiser-Permanente was open to everyone. The idea of a pre-paid medical plan had caught on. In fact a very good natured Sicilian, who genuinely cared about "the little people," and who once raced a produce truck over Southern California's very hazardous "grape-vine highway," felt it was a noble idea. By 1952, labor leader, Joseph T. DeSilva, of Retail Clerks 770, raised $100,000 to establish Kaiser-Permanente in Los Angeles, California.

Physicians, however, by and large favored the system of "fee for service." Blue Cross and similar insurance plans for medical care were put in place. In the fifties a medical consultation costing $25 was considered robbery! $25 paid for 24 hours in a hospital! By the mid-sixties Blue Cross of New York cost slightly less than Blue Cross of California. For New York it took just $32, paid quarterly, for a family of two adults with four children to have just a hospitalization plan. With fee for service, the physician was on his own to serve in his chosen community. After four years of medical school and one year of internship, that commonly included experience in surgery, surgical specialties, internal medicine, obstetrics and pediatrics, one went into general practice, or, went on to try to qualify and be accepted for more training. This usually meant three years of general surgery, and then a year or more training in a surgical specialty. A similar amount of time needed to be invested in internal medicine and then a specialty (e.g. infectious diseases), or, one year of internal medicine and then three years of neurology. Pediatric residency required two consecutive years, with more time in a pediatric specialty. Psychiatric medicine consisted of three consecutive years of psychiatry. Just medical school and a good internship, however, meant the physician could "write his or her own ticket." Parents of "fee for service physicians," just starting out, were boastful. People looked up to their physician, and it wasn't necessary at all to be a specialist as far as the public was concerned. It seemed to everyone that practicing medicine was the ideal profession. Medical practitioners, however, were not businessmen. Being "disease smart" wasn't the same as being "street smart." Doctors were "doctors" and that was just what they were meant to be.

Unfortunately some doctors were unable to fashion themselves that way. They became more business oriented. During the fifties all too many patients, who bought medical insurance, determined also to spoil a good thing. Most often it was the type of patient who wanted to be "screened" for everything! Certain folk chose the "high option." Hearing of laboratory tests they felt they ought to have, they somehow felt "entitled" to these tests. Overlooking the "principle of insurance," they felt since they paid for it, why shouldn't they get tested? Physicians, especially those with good clinical acumen, resisted such patient pressures put upon them and tried to reassure patients without so much lab work, but eventually many doctors simply caved in. Financially focused physicians already offered their patients "lab test menus!" Insurance lobbyist very annoyed with this rising trend complained privately to legislators as well as those of organized medicine. "There were doctors practicing who should not be practicing," they said. They were correct but reasonably it was too late to do anything about it.

Even if a doctor called a case of hemorrhoids "strep throat," if such were agreeable to his patient and the patient didn't complain how would anyone find out? Reportedly a Santa Clara California physician, who owned the pharmacy nearest his office, called virtually all his cases "strep throat!" He had a Spanish speaking practice, was pushing penicillin billing also from his pharmacy to MediCal, California's social welfare plan. The physician, who spoke fluent Spanish was dedicated to "preventing rheumatic heart disease" from striking any patient within his sphere of medical influence. Presumably this was accomplished. Academically such practice redefined absurdity in therapeutics, however, none of his patients complained. He was worshipped instead as a "penicillin god." Taking advantage of the up and coming computer age each case was registered separately as "appropriate treatment for an appropriate condition." His income in the late nineteen sixties was about $70,000 per year, virtually all Medi-Cal (Medicaid). You can be certain the obsessed physician had a lawyer who was in very close touch with a judge who also spoke Spanish.

The Department of Vocational Standards (DVS) received many complaints in California. They ranged from the bewildering to the bizarre. Virtually anything and everything you can imagine became at face value a legitimate request for an investigation! There was no way for such a department to respond to all requests. Having lunch at Posey's restaurant in Sacramento, with Earl Waters, then head of the DVS, some very weird complaints were occasionally related. There was nothing to do but have a chuckle and say, "It's a sick world, and how to 'healers and their patients' get involved in such goings on?" What really was the DVS supposed to do about it?

Nearly all America approved of physicians having a nice home and driving a new car and being able to collect sufficient money to send their children to college. By 1955 certain doctors had already focused on the almighty dollar. A few had "tunnel vision" as they used to say. They were too "focused on the nickel" and nothing else.

In 1960, a professor and chairman of a medical or surgical department in a university teaching center was for the most part delighted to make about $30,000 per year. There was additional income from billings from private practice representing about ten percent of time away from seeing "teaching cases." Sops from pharmaceutical firms were just beginning. The hope was to encourage a less that objective university clinic evaluation of some new drug. It was fortunately a rare professor who went for the money. If he did he was sort of "out of the loop of respect" by medical students that got wind of it.

So called "town and gown battles" became very evident in certain areas. A classic example, when UCLA developed their "ivory tower teaching center," physicians in Beverly Hills were so upset (financially threatened), teaching case material became impeded. Those serving internships in 1958 at UCLA were required to work-up the same clinical teaching case twice for experience while hospitalized ill patients gladly cooperated but suffered déjà vu.

As newly appointed department heads from UCLA swooped into the County Hospital in Torrance California, known then and now as Harbor General Hospital, to assume control of a specialty division exceptional teachers of medicine and pediatrics were brushed aside like Mel Kaplan, MD, internal medicine and Kenneth Zike, MD, pediatrics. In some cases it smacked of arrogant personalities replacing nice people who were also enthusiastic teachers. It seemed sort of obvious the "image of the newly formed institution" was more important than the actual teaching program, or, going further yet whether patients were cared for in the most decent efficient way.

While costs from 1958 to 1961 were "nothing" compared to medical-surgical costs today, even in 1958 emphasis on finance clearly overshadowed medical care. Having just admitted a case of heart failure via the emergency room, the very next morning anxious to check your patient on "dig and merc" you, the "doctor," were surprisingly upstaged! Your patient was being interviewed by a social worker over "property ownership status" should it be necessary to attach a lien. As ordered the nurses had done a good job of propping the struggling patient up to assist his breathing. Valuable information on how much of a diuretic effect had thus far taken place along with quizzing the patient to critically adjust digitalis dosage logically took precedence but never did! Without exception each case was treated as a Los Angeles County "financial emergency!" There's no personal recollection of any exception. More bizarre yet, the patient could not possibly have walked out of the hospital; the rush based on economic fears the patient might have died before the social worker got there to document the information!

For the sociologically complex measurement of costs of medical care from the fifties to just before the "ax" fell during the nineties for instituting managed care, one needs to address units of effort as well as time spent per each task at hand. One wonders too if some narcissistic entitlement syndrome, like "a virus," had previously overcome the entire medical profession! Increasing propaganda designed to convince the American public "over utilization" of high technology instrumentation is necessary, or else you are not receiving the "best medical care," continues on its way to becoming even more of a smashing commercial success.

Public acceptance of "over utilization of medical testing" continues into the 21st century. The trend fails to slow in spite of physician awareness hi-tech instrumentation, thrust upon them through the system, fails to help patients all things considered. Furthermore over utilization comes about not by one doctor's decision but through committee decisions by momes, or greedy business oriented administrators, in concert with insurance providers who never fully understood what physicians are taught to do if those who taught those committee oriented types ever knew in the first place. It's simply a business of making as many bucks as possible on sick patients. How else do you make the hospital payroll? That is a problem.

In spite of amazing medical and surgical accomplishments medical care for the masses worsens for three clear-cut reasons. First physicians are being trained more and more like molecular biologists as if lost in some futuristic dream world that cannot yet be taught. Second is a fixation on "business" in spite of the cost of technology-driven-medical-care exceeding the financial capabilities that man on earth can allow! Third, more patients are being seen in some emergency care center (ER) where stab wounds, bullet wounds and "raving or tripping on various street drugs" are their areas of expertise when such patients "should be seen in the quiet of an appropriate physician's office or via a house call."

As a senior medical student professors encouraged me to become a surgeon, that I was good at it. To this day I've no idea why though some people can remove a sliver from a finger better than someone else. My fascination, however, was about the function of the nervous system particularly the brain or the "mind" (After 40 years I'm still working on it). In America you have the freedom of choice and hopefully the chance to enjoy yourself. Had I been a Soviet medical student at the time of Stalin's dictatorship surgery would have been my profession. Who knows, having skillfully performed some unusual procedure successfully on a celebrity and receiving all kinds of favorable publicity, maybe then one begins to enjoy surgery and thinks, "Uncle Joe was right! On the other hand in the United States you have choice, albeit perhaps not the wisdom to make the best choice. Like your lawyer said, "You married her!" You picked her and she picked you and the marriage turns into a disaster! You then wish you had relied on the wisdom of others with more experience, thinking everything might have worked out, but who on someone else's advice is willing to take such a chance?

Doing some surgery during internship whether enjoying it or not, the first tonsillectomy took only twenty minutes with the patient seated on a chair. Huge tonsils called "kissing tonsils" made the job all the easier. One had to be 15 years or older to have the procedure done in this manner utilizing a local anesthetic. You were instructed *Not To Bother The Patient's Carotid Arteries* and I meticulously obeyed those instructions! Having practiced this "art" over the years imagining time involved, the procedure, "Tonsils in; Tonsils out," should by this time take about six minutes!

Why is it then a whole hour is scheduled for a simple tonsillectomy in an outpatient wing of any major medical center or hospital? Why not 30 minutes? Why not do four patients in that hour?

As an intern it was fun to order a "tray" and fix an umbilical hernia in a few minutes for merely a "thanks Doc." Why during the nineteen nineties did an insurance carrier have to pay just the surgeon's fee of $2500 (!) for fixing an umbilical hernia for a close friend of mine in Los Altos Hills, California? With that "tray" I'd have fixed it for $100 right in his home! That way, had there been an unlikely post-op infection, a few dollars worth of penicillin would have taken care of it! There was no risk in someone's home of a "hospital environment penicillin resistant staph-aureus." Such a "hospital related complication;" the treatment cost alone for I.V. antibiotics has in my own experience been as high as $20,000!

As for "cataract removal," it was a dead animal's eye for practice in a lab. It wasn't easy. On the other hand I've been told that graduates of the "cataract school of India" go village to village removing cataracts at the proper time needing about 20 minutes for each case.

By the late fifties cataract removal cost $300 in San Francisco California. In 1962, during my residency at UCSF I dash across town to see a cataract patient (my dad). He tells me the charge is $700! He's visibly upset about the charge. Looking at the surgery schedule board it's shows his Stanford eye-surgeon has several cataract cases scheduled for that morning.

As a neurologist or ophthalmologist, utilizing dim lighting rather than dilating the pupils with local medication, it takes little effort to visualize the retina, optic nerve head and macula. If "seeing-in" is easy, "seeing-out" for the patient is easier yet (!), so why during the nineteen-eighties are so many patients having cataract procedures? Is it just a way of making money? Could that be it? Checking on the economics of the matter Medicare during the eighties is paying $1327 for removal of one cataract and a synthetic lens being put in its' place. But, patients tell me the eye surgeon's fee goes beyond what Medicare pays and even exceeds $2000! Allotted time for out patient cataract surgery is sometimes scheduled for two hours, or way more time than is typically necessary. If the procedure is not performed in the ophthalmologist's office herein suggests "a cooperative plan" to obtain more money from Medicare to meet local hospital needs. The actual task typically takes much less than one hour unless you are just going to admit the "Hindus are better at it than American ophthalmologists."

One day getting an urgent call from a hospital nurse working in-hospital out-patient surgery she tells me the ophthalmologist fails to show until ten minutes into the second hour scheduled. As a result the patient, a rough, tough fellow from Midland Texas, demonstrates his anger to the nurse with a blood pressure of 230/150! Knowing the patient for years and that his blood pressure is typically about 160/90 since he's nearly always angry about something - and usually with good reason - I reassure the nurse and the procedure is postponed. Two days later checking the patient his BP is where it usually is and a few days later his cataract surgery is a complete success.

About the same time I had several patients who had come to America from New Delhi India.

One family ran a leather business successfully but his wife had convulsive seizures for which she was given sleeping pills and her seizure symptoms were becoming more violent. With simply a good medical history and a clinical neurological exam that was negative, and with a bit of therapeutic luck, I placed the patient very gingerly on primidone (Mysoline). As a result she never had another spell and to be ever so careful about "costs," she was followed without any lab tests whatsoever and without electroencephalography. In addition, since the medication increased the requirement for a little extra folic acid vitamin in the diet it appeared her Hindu dietary habits over time were more than adequate. She always looked well and seemed happy and full of energy, hardly the picture of any form of anemia. The whole family was delighted "mother was at last seizure free." (What a nice grateful family and the treatment so simple).

The seizure patient's husband became my patient since he was a "mahatma Ghandi freedom fighter" entitled to a stipend yearly the only covenant he had to submit evidence of an annual physical exam. I noted he had a small cataract. Finally it was "ripe for removal." In other words, although the patient could still see out, I could no longer see his eye grounds. A round trip flight to New Delhi was $700 with a 14-day stay. Removal of his cataract in India was to cost $25 U.S! The implantation of a synthetic lens was $100. U.S. for a total cost of $825 Understandably most all Americans, especially given a rather long list of real albeit unlikely complications, were too leery to opt for cataract removal, India-style, following say a one-week tour of India. Furthermore, by the nineteen-eighties, the strain financially on Medicare was so high what you saved the system having your cataract removed in the U.S., the outrageous price notwithstanding, was relatively speaking, insignificant. It all depended really on how badly you wanted to visit India and if you could be convinced the Hindus knew what they were doing.

Acquiring good help is always a challenge for any employer. Those evaluating applicants for medical school face the same situation. In the fifties sons of doctors who wanted to become doctors are clearly a best bet, particularly if such an applicant is one of those "A-students." For the remainder of applicants the one-on-one interview on especially "why" one wants to become a physician is extremely critical for decision-making, more so than straight A-grades. Back then only five percent or so of medical school classes are female simply because the masses are accustomed to physicians being men! By the nineteen-eighties and nineties computer profiling surely enters the big picture with grades listed on a computer being ever so important. Medical school classes nowadays often consist of more women than men. Why not? Einstein and Newton clearly are in the "male category" but this is not a good basis for any valid argument women are not equal to men. For instance there's Madame Curie who shared one Nobel Prize in physics then went on to win one in chemistry entirely on her own. Only Linus Pauling is given the edge winning two unshared Nobel Prizes. Both men and women are equally able to succeed whether in pure science or as physicians. It's important, however, that a woman physician with special attributes not dress like a waitress at Hooters if she plans to see male patients or women attracted to women.

Medical school applicants today are apt to be much less naive than thirty years ago but being less naive is not the same as predicting you are going to be a good doctor. Sadly, many doctors today are unaware of the difference between being a good physician and what too many have turned out to be. Some teachers aren't good physicians or good instructors either. This seems true wherever education is so important conceivably in very many fields. An inclination to demonstrate no "good will" to inspire the student is also part of the overall problem! Instead of teaching it's "Look it up in some journal and report to me in the morning!" (My professors happily were not that way. Time was not wasted when something could be taught quickly.)

Expectancy the past 40 years ranges from being satisfied with a nice living to becoming very greedy or, sadly, to have to work for one of so many health maintenance organizations (HMO's). In these situations pay is so much per patient or so much per task at hand and definitely not, even time-wise, on the doctor's own terms. Nowadays one hears of physicians, even specialists who after all their training just quit! It's tragic. On the other hand, some with great patience, motivation and talent navigate to the top of the "U.S. pyramid system." Others fold, become discouraged, depressed, resort to alcohol or mind altering drugs and the suicide rate goes up. For those somehow "cut out for the game of major money," they're the ones who maintain close ties to hospital needs. Both doctor and hospital collect inordinate sums of money proposing and doing tests and treatments even detrimental to patients. For example: patient "G.T." DOB 8/31/67, Sherman Medical Claim (Connecticut Gen. Life Ins.), Fedex Grp. Plan #07559070486-235639, Inv. #3322384.

During 1966 Edward R. Annis, MD, president of the American Medical Association, pleads with the U.S. Congress NOT to pass Medicare, prophetic that "money will take over!" All pleading falling on deaf ears, Medicare passes. By 1967 medical and surgical treatment billings, as physician Annis said prophetically, are already on the rise. "Capitation, along the lines of medical-surgical competition adopted by the Canadian system of medical care delivery is brushed aside.

The "DeBakey Plan," a visionary proposal by the famed heart and vascular surgeon pioneer for regional centers for cancer, stroke and heart disease, actually part of the idealism of President Lyndon Johnson's "Great Society," was quickly rejected by the political arm of organized medicine. The impact of this rejection was so great that an extremely well trained neurologist, formerly married then divorced from a daughter of a past president of the California Medical Association simply had quite enough and committed suicide. He was UCSF trained and then practicing in San Rafael, California. He was also a friend of mine.

"Family physicians" were not about to be upstaged. What's wrong with "mediocre care" anyway? It has been pretty well established about half of all presentations to physician's offices consisted of anxiety states. "Family physicians, however, were not trained nearly well enough in psychiatric medicine to recognize or allay anxiety. It has also been recognized this major deficiency sometimes led to unnecessary "exploratory" surgery. There were good "GPs," however, who naturally had good surgical skills. Realizing their error upon exploration they told their patient they made a great mistake. The GP explained, "Jane, I'm distressed to tell you this but you did not have an enlarged cystic ovary as I thought. All you really needed was a "good laxative!" The reply for such professional honesty was, "Really? Well, doctor, that's all right and I'm glad to know I'm okay. You were genuinely concerned for me and that's what counts and I'm happy my ovary is fine. The procedure was as much my fault as yours so when do I get out of here?" The neighbors grew to like the doctor more. Why? It was because of honesty. Furthermore it was resolved that next time a laxative might be tried first!

Ten years prior to a period during the late nineteen-seventies many physicians in private practice, particularly solo docs, began to feel the HMO known as Kaiser-Permanente was not so bad after all. Kaiser by then had attracted many able physicians and surgeons, all getting paid with no hassle, and, with a one-month yearly vacation when their worries about patients could in large part be left behind.

The political arm of organized medicine, however, was unwilling to even imagine "one big Kaiser plan in the U. S." There was also the threat of that "single payer" Canadian Plan, working in those days extremely very well up north. Canadian doctors didn't care about becoming rich off medical care. They wanted to be happy. They were happy! The American counterpart was becoming progressively more disgruntled and unhappy.

Obfuscation proved necessary along with the propaganda that the Canadian Plan was "socialized medicine." It never was! The glittering generalities of advertising portrayed the US health care system as the greatest in the world!   Those of the AMA with experience and wisdom, like Dwight Wilbur, spoke out reflecting on the "Flexner Report of 1909." Mindful another such report might be justified as how best to educate medical students to become good doctors, he emphasized in the mean time "catastrophic insurance." The rising cost of coming technology was obviously going to prove to be too much to afford. "Fee for service medicine" was still working pretty well though fees were bound to become more difficult to collect as costs increased. Investigative and repair techniques were improving in conjunction with high technology but, without catastrophic insurance, it was surely going to be a case of best medical care eventually just for the rich. Political emphasis of necessity was in support of increasingly expensive sophisticated technology. In our capitalistic society employment was of major importance at the highest level of political thinking. AMA former president Dwight Wilbur of San Francisco was also concerned about his son, Dwight Wilbur MD internist in Sacramento's future practicing medicine. I first met them in the Wilbur home in San Francisco when young Dwight and I were in the sixth grade at US Grant elementary school in 1941, and years later when we both attended Lowell High School. Unlike Dwight Jr., it had never entered my mind for a second that I would one day become a physician.

On the other hand, why couldn't everyone have learned to simply use an abacus? How difficult was the math? Instead bigwigs of organized medicine met with various folk, nostalgic for the days of Thomas John Watson Sr. and Jr. of IBM, to develop a computerized system of billing that was to become a specialty within itself! Was high technology really necessary for this? Over "gin rummy," after a few drinks in some hotel, there began to be devised a "coding system," whereby only a main frame computer was able to store all the gibberish, (a normal human brain would logically flush most of it out). Eventually, some 2,500 relative value numbers were fed into a storage and retrieval (RVS) system! Seminars were held, then more seminars proved necessary, in order to train office managers so a physician could get paid without committing fraud! Any mistake, on any one of over a thousand different insurance forms, translated automatically into a "money making strategic-delay for the payer," which obviously was part of the whole plan that favored the insurance companies!

Amidst payment delays, confusion, harassment and frustration, computer fraud (white-collar crime) was assured. Patient's visits were "timed." If the intent was to make some physicians work for nothing, then what ensued was not only immoral and dishonest in terms of business ethics, but, along with murder, was classifiable under "sins that cry out to heaven!" Doctor and staff became "thugs so as to survive!" Juggling of recorded procedures, and time spent with patients to pick the most reasonable "code number," became the game! But, as aforementioned, the whole gig was "very good for employment," and again "employment was the most important at the highest level of political thinking." And so for the sake of employment the real agony began!

For listing a "diagnosis on a certain form," the RVS "numbers game" (racket) was to prove more asinine yet! Medical societies had selected physicians for "peer review." Young doctors called on older physicians who had practiced for years. A physician-henchman informed a practicing internist he was not to make a judgment call on an insurance form like "chronically depressed!" It didn't matter that the impression was absolutely correct. It had to be a printed diagnosis clearly within the specialty that was programmed into the computer! Only a "psychiatrist was 'computer authorized to list depression' as a primary diagnosis." And then, even if it was too soon to say, the psychiatrist had to list depression as "endogenous," or "situational," or "double," (both) or part of a bi-polar mood disorder. The computer was totally unable to "think about, or log the truth." Billings kept going through as "bi-polar" when in truth it was discovered, "bi-polar really meant cocaine or amphetamines in the morning and booze, or heroin, in the evening!" It made no difference so long as one avoided confusing the computer. Any correction made was guaranteed to stop an insurance-payer in its tracks and the physician might "never get paid!" Non-physician business-educated nurses with computer experience were hired to process huge stacks of forms for an insurance carrier perhaps two days per week! As a result gross over-payments involving scads of unnecessary tests slipped through while certain physicians, mostly solo docs still trying desperately to survive in spite of the "system," were put through the "tortures of hell in terms of payment starvation for doing the right thing."

The Industrial Revolution was not a "revolution" in that it came about so gradually. Furthermore there was a real need for a cotton gin. The U.S. needed a railroad to connect its two coasts. Machines were often welcomed and given affectionate names like, "Charlie." By comparison the technological revolution has been properly named, since it has jolted everyone. In medicine for 20 years or so it has been "CT-PET-MRI scanomania!" Thrust upon the masses has been the "lap top computer," introduced in 1981. Sadly, as instrumentation in general has increased it has supplanted the all-important "careful medical history" (and physical exam). Unnecessary treatments including surgical procedures have become more and more prevalent.

For the storage of volumes of data along with quick retrieval and the performing of stochastic algorhythyms (the human genome project) there's nothing that can match the speedy computer. On the other hand, for references, the Columbia Encyclopedia is much too convenient to ever be replaced and to me it seems senseless to try. In addition it seems a trifle obtuse to me to convey the notion it's easier to teach a first grader usefully as the child gazes at some computer screen. Testing on any subject, for that matter, is best by way of an essay examination! It may be more labor intensive to correct, but if the student really knows nothing, then he or she cannot even compose a sentence about the subject matter, and both examiner and student clearly know where they stand. An essay format also deprives any examiner of the odd satisfaction of asking what is all too often amusingly referred to as a "trick question." A computer of course can easily correct a multiple-choice or true-false test enabling the teacher to get paid for doing next to nothing once the computer program is in place. Regardless the computer does offer a partial solution where there is a shortage of teachers and too large a class of students. The ideal is a small number of students, an interesting teacher and more personalization. Granted, it's a big order, but it is an order that better be met! It's not being met as yet!

By the nineteen eighties it became well known insurance companies bought into much high-tech equipment. Privatization became a pattern and thus making a substantial profit took on greater importance than simply taking the time to talk to a patient, and to have the patient respond to the ever important line of questioning. Scanners de-emphasized the interpersonal relationship between doctor and patient that was to bring out a quintessential medical history that led to the correct judgment call for the patient. As years passed one witnessed ideal patient care relegated for the sake of financial profits. The pushing of expensive technology was for technocrat's sake.

For example for the many years Transamerica-Occidental managed Medicare in southern California allegiance to supporting technology seemed first and foremost. Should their reply be one of "totally false" to such allegations then why were salesmen, representing for instance Beckman Instruments, calling upon neurologists to lease "brain-map-machines" for office use for about $700 per month? Why were the same neurologists informed Medicare would pay $400 for each such test representing 80% of what Medicare "allowed?" Just ten such "maps" per month meant $4000 from Medicare! The striking fact was that the test, fraught with artifacts, was of limited value, particularly in an office setting except as a flashy scheme to "razzle-dazzle" patients. The test was developed for recording evoked potentials from visual, hearing as well as pain stimuli, for evaluating severely brain-injured patients! An absence of evoked auditory potentials meant certain brain-stem connections were not functioning, hardly the outpatient sort of situation! What was behind Medicare's "approval to pay such moneys" and encourage "office use for such equipment?"

At the same time Transamerica indicated Medicare was not going to be cheated! During the nineteen-eighties a "Transamerica-Occidental Medicare 'Integrity' Handbook" arrived in physician's offices. The apparent purpose was to chide the doctor for cheating Medicare. At the very top of one (mine) personal "computerized cheating list," the most egregious overcharge for the year was $80: house-call for Earl S., Corona de Mar, California, summoned there when the patient fell unconscious to the floor! Driving 11 miles round trip from my office to evaluate this patient for a charge of $80 didn't seem "excessive." What kind of "Medicare integrity was that?"

It occurred perhaps that those involved in the grand scheme of things programmed the Medicare computer not to look upon housecalls favorably. A house call was identified by the computer as a threat interfering with nearby emergency room and hospital "business!" Again it was a matter of employing as many people as possible whether those involved were doing the right thing or what was necessary or not. Consumer advocates had fallen prey to corporate America. The ill patients, and his or her family, were gradually not going to be able to have a preference in such a predicament, their only hope being the physician willing to make the house call, and then the physician was supposedly "cheating the business arrangements with Medicare!" That's what the integrity handbook alleged.

Earl S., my house call to be patient was referred to me by a former osteopath who came west in 1929 to become the first physician in Laguna Beach, California. His name was Vincent "Hap" (for happy) Carroll who became officially a California MD in 1962. Vince was not only actress Betty Davis' favorite doctor, but also the favorite as well of Mrs. Meifert Irvine. When "Hap, the osteopath" delivered Betty Davis' baby, rumors flew all over the place MD gynecologists hoped something would go wrong! When everything went perfectly well, jealousy being what it is, there was tremendous disappointment. Because of Vincent Carroll, Mrs. Irvine donated the land for the building of South Coast Hospital on a hill at the south end of Laguna Beach. Well, Earl S. just like many others who settled many years ago in Orange County, California, were, for whatever reason "osteopathically oriented." Doc Carroll knew Earl and his family well enough to know they had no desire for fancy high technology procedures. In addition, Earl and his family were adamant against Earl being hospitalized, if there was any way this could be avoided. To oblige everyone Earl remained my out-patient house-call for nine consecutive years. During that time he did require from four to seven medications-a nineteen eighties drug bill of some $400 per month-for cardio-vascular and other problems. It took those nine long years for "management at Hoag Hospital in Newport Beach to finally catch another big fish!" I was in Cabo San Lucas on vacation. As a result Earl received the "medical work-up of his entire lifetime," and for what? For money: Medicare money and some of Earls'! Earl was then introduced to their fairly new profit-making, high employment "Alzheimer's Program." Going along with the jargon of Ross Perot running for president of the U.S. you could "hear the sucking sound as Medicare money at last was being drained at Earl's expense. It was an apparent case of making up for lost profit-making-time. One was able to estimate the housecalls, that in every case obviated the need to dial 911, or pay for ambulance rides then hospital work-ups typically always "gilding the lily," over nine consecutive years, saved America's Medicare money- pool of about $400,000! That was just "for 'one patient' named, "Earl S."

Way beyond any solo-physician's control surprising things can and do happen. Occasionally it's expected. When what happens becomes unbelievable it can become bewildering! Is it conceivable that suddenly the financial aspects of medical practice can revert back to 1938 when so many doctors took care of patients for nothing? Is it not far beyond the imagination when the economic practices of the very medical center where you spent four years as a medical student and three more years in residency suddenly threaten to put you, their product, out of business? Is it possible chancellors and deans that manage medical centers to train doctors going into private practice no longer see the "big picture," or even care?

During the "AIDs epidemic" of the nineteen eighties AIDs patient' demands, and ultimately political-economic responses to those demands to manage the problem with all it's far reaching complications, led to the bankruptcy of many small insurance carriers. In short AIDs created a medical-political-insurance disaster that cascaded to adversely affect many innocent patients in need of medical care for "other ills," along with some way to pay for their medical needs even though they didn't have AIDs. After all there were other diseases needing medical as well as surgical attention besides AIDs.

As if the cost of medicines to treat AIDs was not enough, it was just by chance I learned first hand of two payments for intracranial AIDs complications neurosurgery at my alma mater,

UCSF, for $125,000 and $135,000 respectively received on the very same day! In other words payments received in that department in one day totaled one quarter of a million dollars reportedly for two (?) AID case surgeries! Within one year six patients seen in my office in Laguna Beach California, 440 miles from San Francisco loaded with AIDs patients discovered their completely paid-up medical insurance plans are worthless! All six of their insurance carriers had declared bankruptcy! In other words premium moneys my patients had paid into their plans had been all used up substantially (!) for treating AIDs patients! Two of my six patients required hospitalization. Like many things the AIDs crisis could have been ameliorated by closing the gay bath houses of San Francisco much sooner, and country wide by allocating essential funding to blood banks (!) to immediately improve their testing procedures. In addition, an effort by the American Medical Association to get information to the nation's physicians regarding blood bank practices would have helped a great deal. In complete opposition as to what was previously taught to medical students and doctors, it was too late discovered less need to use blood so generously! What most physicians finally learned by 2002 could have and should have been known by nearly all practicing physicians by the middle of the nineteen eighties!

One bankrupted carrier covered employees that installed interiors for corporate jets in Huntington Beach, California. Another example to be specific was "Ace" of Chicago, Illinois. The female patient covered by Ace was a goner without hospitalization. It was 1:00 A.M. when I reached her hospital room and just in the nick of time. She recognized me then emerged slowly from her bed constantly repeating senseless words, stared vacantly, stiffened and fell "like a lamp post." Luckily I grabbed her head just before it struck the floor preventing, conceivably, an intracranial hematoma (more expense!). After 13 rather severe seizures at intervals she finally stabilized completely on well-shaken primidone (Mysoline) suspension administered via a naso-gastric tube. A pretty lady, formerly a bathing suit model living in Hawaii, she had unwittingly put herself in harm's way. Joining her wealthy girl friend with marital difficulties they both took off in her girl friend's Rolls-Bentley Corniche to enjoy a "two week toot." The car made it without a scratch; but one of those girls almost didn't. She made it learning what too much alcohol can cause in some people. In her case it was "repeated seizure symptom activity that could have been fatal if not checked in time."

Not happy working for nothing it was time to call "Ace" of Chicago to ask higher management if they couldn't please pay me "something." The reply, "Doctor I would like to pay you, however we just issued our final check in the amount of six figures and we are bankrupt!" "Was that check to U.C. San Francisco for some AIDs patient's surgery?" "I'm sorry but where our check was sent has to remain confidential." The grateful patient, robbed of her insurance coverage, nevertheless, paid my bill of about $900 in monthly installments over the next year. She also paid the hospital bill. Both doctor and the hospital were in luck in view of her insurance carrier's bankruptcy. This gesture to pay was because her life was saved and she knew it. Otherwise, for those of us who work for a living the philosophical adjustment to pay again, when you're paid up medical insurance policy suddenly has lost its ability to help you one iota, may be too much. As a result neither the managing physician nor hospital gets paid, especially in view of the bankruptcy of both the medical care insurance carrier and perhaps the patient as well.

What needs to be gotten across to the gay community, celebrities raising funds, lawmakers in congress and those with influence in the White House is that there are other diseases that need to be addressed, their puzzles solved with funding, besides AIDs! Personally I have never known of anyone who suffered with arthritis, with multiple sclerosis, with multiple myeloma, with Parkinson's disease that would not have been more than happy to use a condom (the same applies to a sterile needle) if that prevented what those patients disease-wise had to endure. "Everybody desires to have love and love is wonderful but you shouldn't welcome in a serious disease going for it!" With syphilis also dramatically on the rise among gay, bisexual, and other men who have sex with men (MSM) it is estimated HIV transmission is increased two to five times! A saying long before the age of penicillin, "Five minutes with Venus then a life time with mercury," may have instilled caution back then but nothing seems to work now.

Someone of course will deny it but by the nineteen nineties many doctors who had pledged allegiance to the political arm of organized medicine realized medical care in America, good and bad, was being delivered somewhat short of moral excellence. What helped signal America's medical delivery system's eventual doom was a bank assuming forceful money collection responsibilities for medical centers as well as many out lying hospitals. Making matters worse for those suffering and needing hospitalization there was no confident way provided to determine "costs in advance for either in-patient or out patient procedures, let alone required hospitalizations." The biggest part of the mystery was what one out of hundreds of insurance plans might pay with everything less than perfectly programmed into computers. Nobody in a hospital seemed anxious to make as much as a telephone call to Blue Cross or anyone else. The cost was whatever amount could be weaseled out of your plan and after that what could be weaseled out of you! And that was the intent from the beginning of any patient's cost inquiry.

When insurance plans paid less than expected secretaries for specialists in medical centers and general hospitals were offered incentives, actually commissions, for collecting all amounts unpaid often constituting staggering surgical and hospital costs. A second mortgage of a home was not unusual to prevent or relieve the hopeless agony of persistent computerized billings via a depersonalized, commercialized system that typically included over utilization of test equipment and therefore more than necessary medical center personnel.

There were even substantial payment demands for a pharmacist standing watch over a ward. Patient medications ordered and recorded in the chart, as if physicians and nurses on that service didn't know what they were doing, were reviewed and checked by a pharmacist! Exorbitant extra sums collected there was a rationale by medical center management about the need for extra money to be poured into medical student teaching programs, even though it was obvious too many doctors were continually being produced each year! Too many "tests to be sure," when logical expectancy dictated many of the tests were unnecessary, as well as a feeling on the part of many they had not received their money's worth, became the perception of many "victims of hospitalization" by the late nineteen eighties.

Countrywide some 15% of the U.S. gross domestic product was being utilized for medical care! Furthermore Congress which controls money seemed unaware that medical care for most had deteriorated, desirous of hearing only of spectacular things being done. Astonishingly there were those associated with stock and bond investment firms who felt America was still under-medicated! All this was happening as costs of medications skyrocketed while a great many patients were taking, objectively speaking, medications they didn't really need! The 10percent of 1.42 trillion dollars, for cost of medicines during 2002, incurred on the ability of all too many to buy food!

Having reviewed some of the history of finance in the US reveals, without a Federal Reserve System with 12 regional banks to reserve and discount member banks, our country would have plunged into financial disarray early in the 20th century! Towards the latter part of the 20th century various regional banks had taken charge of collecting medical bills. Armored cars were regularly seen making hospital rounds. The cost of care rose to astronomical amounts!" Solutions to problems were left to each state having their peculiar set of governing laws. Organized medicine displayed no sympathy for so-called "working poor," and did its best to dodge the issue, finally winding up holding "a tiger by the tail." Organized medicine was nevertheless appalled by any idea of a federally organized medical delivery system! In retrospect it brought to mind the newspaper comic strip decades ago called "Smokey Stover," by Rube Goldberg. Smokey had so many stove pipes with dimensional differences, angles and twists leading from point-A to the flue, point-B; when he fixed one problem he simply created another. Laughingly you were reminded of "political reforms" and what those engaged in politics face when the answer is, "there is no answer!" "Turning over a new leaf," was on the mind of Congressman John Moss 30 years ago (!) but when will America be willing to do that?

Selfish ambition within the medical profession remains largely the blame for America's political health care predicament. Those in organized medicine along with those ascending to power fail to show consideration for idealistic physicians willing to address the "needs" of sick patients for much less money than those kinds of physicians deserve. Consideration isn't shown for patients unable to afford sophisticated technological tests, expensive ER visits or hospitalizations, let alone the staggering cost of so many kinds of highly advertised medications. The power of television drives too many of the public into an exaggerated need for some new medicine. It may be ridiculous but it seems an inescapable fact.

No one knows the whole story but hearsay has it former California Governor Ronald Reagan just barged ahead and cut welfare and medical services. Part of the record reveals that MediCal (Medicaid of CA.) was declared bankrupt three weeks prior to Ronald Reagan being re-elected to a second term as governor. Of interest Ronald Reagan was never told of this until after his re-election! Behind the scenes it was organized medicine that engineered the bankruptcy. This gesture denied payments of hundreds of thousands of dollars to physicians who had already performed services and also had all their forms correctly submitted and approved! In other words it was "a case of political doctors cheating practicing doctors!" Lobbyists and campaign politicians were told not to tip off the governor and keep their mouths shut knowing Ronald Reagan would "hit the roof" and oppose any ploy to deny physicians what they had already earned with "fees way below normal charges!" He had nothing to do with any of this except take the blame. At first I blamed him then found out Ronald Reagan was never told. (Iran-Contra also comes to mind speaking of Reagan. When he said he never knew it was because he didn't.)

Reagan was extremely fair-minded. He listened carefully and made decisions based on right versus wrong. Never mind the votes. He just didn't care if you voted for him or you didn't. I believe he was literally dragged into politics and "votes" later had nothing to do with his decisions. As a Republican Reagan heeded the call of Ralph Nader's favorite feisty insurance commissioner of Pennsylvania, Herbert Dennenberg. In the sixties Mr. Dennenberg publicly exposed Blue Cross executives for concentrating on personal financial gain above everything else. What Blue Cross was supposed to do for members was secondary. That such a prediction was prophetic was verified in the late nineteen-eighties when Governor Mario Cuomo of New York, embarrassed by scandal after scandal involving Blue Cross of New York, saw to it the head of Blue Cross was fired. During the nineteen nineties notices to California physicians were sent warning beware of fraudulent Blue Cross activities. Why hadn't organized medicine's representatives stepped in many years ago to prevent or correct fraudulent Blue Cross wrong doings? Was organized medicine benefiting? What prevented such action over the course of four decades? Now, for the 12/4/02 issue of USA Today, Bruce Bodaken, CEO, Blue Shield of California says to Julie Appleby, "California has long been a trendsetter for the rest of the country. Now is the time for us to lead the rest of the country toward achieving 'universal coverage.' It is a daunting challenge, but we can't wait." (What are the chances of insurance companies allowing a single payer plan instead of continuing to endure thuggery inherent in our present system?)

During the late forties President Harry Truman used the bully pulpit and declared a national health plan for the United States; a plan that included everyone as the only "civilized approach becoming a nation like the United States." There was little or no support from organized medicine. Famous actor Edward G. Robinson supported the idea but why would he care?. He had money to pay his medical bills. His best friend, Jacob "Jack" Karp, last president of Paramount Studios before the Gulf -Western merger, supported the idea. Why? Jack Karp had money to pay his family's medical expenses. Why would these two famous and quite wealthy men care about others who might not be able to afford decent medical care? Why wouldn't the politicians of the American Medical Association see things that way? Jack Karp, head of the legal department then comptroller of Paramount Studios, who paid Ronald Reagan's salary, sat me down one day with his son Bob (who years later became a highly respected cardiovascular surgeon), and carefully described a sensible two-tiered health plan. That was 1955, our second year at UCSF medical school. It sounded so logical and reasonable it seemed such a two-tiered arrangement would simply come about. In fact Bob and I expected it. For patients that could afford to pay for extra medical advice it was all right for them to go ahead and do it! Now, 47 years later, America's health delivery has gotten instead more completely screwed up! A top of the line heart surgeon like Dr. Karp must pay $180,000 a year in 2003 for a malpractice policy! Where did this expectation originate that everyone who graduates from medical school can surgically repair the heart? (And Medicare policy has things so structured it prevents Bill Gates and Warren Buffet from purchasing a private room in a hospital unless they have a documented "acute condition." Even if either man purchased the hospital for personal reasons, that very hospital would lose its peer review while being investigated for irregularities.)

Dr. Karp retired in 2000 after 17years head of heart surgery at the University of Chicago. Recently I spoke with two nurses that missed him as head of their department. I retired from active practice in 1998 no longer able to treat patients without intrusions in solo private practice. Both of us look back knowing how much room there's been for improvement over the past four decades; also knowing no doctor or group of doctors can do much of anything about it.

President Bill Clinton introduced a national health plan before the US Congress early during his first term. Since it seemed insurmountable to suddenly start over, e.g. turn over a new leaf, the Clinton Plan meant definite improvements for everybody! It was as if the sun had finally come out after years of darkness!. Within days, however, the AMA delivered their printed booklet with their interpretation of such a Plan to all the nation's physicians, members or not! Their message as: "It's too complicated-The Clinton Plan won't work!" Unlike the Clinton Plan that was not hard to understand, it was virtually impossible to understand what exactly the AMA was implying in their printed rejection of that plan.

Dan Rostenkowski, Chicago, Illinois, chairman of ways and means, the most powerful position probably in the United States Congress, who during 1983 was noted for helping keep our Social Security Plan solvent, publicly indicated the Clintons had chosen the right course and he was very supportive. Then, as if lightning struck, someone figured a way to "neutralize Dan Rostenkowski!" On television a tall young lawyer who apparently represented the pharmaceutical cartel, excuse me, "industry." told everyone who tuned in, "No one is above the law!" What a coincidence! "Rosty," who had served his community very well for many years was on the verge of being jailed apparently because someone in his congressional office had converted postage stamps into money! The amount of money questionably was perhaps equivalent to costs for 24 hours worth of mostly unnecessary tests in some emergency room.

Doesn't it seem unusual for a "politician from Chicago" needing a few extra bucks to have to resort to selling postage stamps to get it? Wouldn't there be a better less complicated and quicker way? Talk about Jimmy Hoffa being railroaded, the chairman of the most powerful U.S. congressional office gets sentenced to 17 months! It's a wonderment how someone from Al Capone's hometown could be jailed because he's associated with someone who sold postage stamps for money!

For all of Capone's reported misbehavior historical accounts reveal he was given a sentence served in Alcatraz for income tax evasion. Undoubtedly he would have been sentenced sooner and more harshly had "Big Al" come out for a federal health plan! Meyer Lansky certainly had more than enough brains to formulate a universal health care system pocketing a little on the side and if he did America would now be ten times better off! Maybe some of the wrong people have been investigated with some wrongfully sent to the penitentiary!

It's 2003 with the U.S. involved in one zany domestic or global situation after another flaunting our successes and military might worldwide. The number one super-power and richest nation in the world continues to elect a Congress that unabashedly leaves 45 million US citizens without any medical care coverage whatever! Congress, the insurance lobby and the pharmaceutical lobby apparently believe balloons don't pop regardless of how much "hot air" you blow into them! Propaganda says the United States sponsors the best health care delivery system in the world. Test it out! Get sick here, then in Canada. You'll discover the Canadians offer a much nicer and efficient plan with happier physicians and happier patients. Of course if you never become ill you will continue to believe what you want to believe. Stay healthy!

"The Canadian Plan is not socialized medicine!" It's very competitive but with "CAPITATION." The Canadian single payer Plan with one standard payment form would be ideal for Cuba as well. Fidel Castro, Jesuit educated lawyer knows of all the problems inherent in America's health care system as not fulfilling his ideal for the Cuban people. You may not like Castro, and you may have good reasons, but do you think he's stupid? Think again. America continues with a health delivery system that "hits a man when he's down." There must be a better way to practice medicine! Strangely enough most everyone who talks health plan in America speaks disparagingly of the Canadian Plan as socialized medicine, when the "socialism is right here in America" and it isn't working altogether very well.

America's health delivery system continues as a pyramid system. This includes payment of fees to physicians. Those at or near the top of the pyramid who maximize the use of hospital services (the utilization of sophisticated high tech equipment) are paid way too much. Those at the middle of the pyramid gradually sliding downward, steadfastly trying to the right thing struggling through each day" get paid less. For dedicated poorly business like physicians who nevertheless enjoy community practice they are destined to remain at the bottom of the pyramid, unless they cave in and accept some financial scheme in conjunction with their local hospital. Survival in solo practice seems nowadays out of the question. Paying overhead beginning practice and paying down accumulated debt from training isn't possible. The concept of retirement for any community practitioner is a dream not to be fulfilled. The reward for all the years of education is soon bound to be "a sandwich sign that reads 'will check your pulse and blood pressure for food'." All this as those that continue to teach medical students to produce more doctors from medical schools retire with living wills that last till the day they die which all adds up to more money typically than their families even need.

Of course it's the so-called "third house that pulls the purse strings in Washington. It is presumed that eventually everyone will cave in to a federally formed medical care plan "with strict pricing for all procedures." The nation's economic picture will make it happen. It's a matter of time and how long do you have to live to experience it? President Harry Truman urges the citizens of the US to "head in such a 'civilized' direction in 1946!" President Bill Clinton directs the citizens of the US that way in 1993. Ten years pass and it gets worse by the month..

The Canadian Plan takes something like nine percent of the Canadian gross national product as compared to nearly 15% of the GNP in the US. The Canadian Plan incorporates the quintessential feature "defined as a uniform per capita payment or fee." In other words "no matter how great you think you are, and even if you 'are,' and, you 'can' walk on water," you only receive so much remuneration per patient evaluation or procedure you perform but "you do get paid!"

When one considers free enterprise and "capitalism" is there anything more mind boggling than macro (global) economics? As consumer demands in the U.S. shrink a bit one looks for instance at the worlds' number two economy, Japan. Japan, with less revenue from the U.S. is in more trouble with "flat growth" for over more than two consecutive years. Output, prices, jobs, profits, incomes, business investment, consumption as well as tax revenue are all down in Japan! Oil prices, however, are up and Japan is 100% dependent, just as Japan was were before WW II! Confidence in the future is compromised; Japanese are saving as much as 30% of household income while the U.S. saves essentially nothing! Japan, regardless having 2.5 trillion $U.S. loaned out as of 2001 nevertheless faces regional and national debt reportedly in the amount equal to 140% of each year's gross domestic product! Bankers make esoteric estimates Japan's wealth collapses by 18 trillion $U.S while at the same time U.S. wealth is "up" 22 trillion $U.S! If that's really the case why can't the U.S. easily afford a medical care delivery plan for all of its citizens? Does anyone understand this? Is there an accountant that understands all this? Can Alan Greenspan explain all this? If during 2002 America is "up" 22 trillion $US, can't the wealthy of America afford to help 45 million of its citizens have some access to reasonable medical care by 2003?

Alan Greenspan, chairman of the Fed "understands." One is persuaded to think former president Bill Clinton possessed the intellect to understand all this yet there must be some lack of understanding from statistical mis-sense. If not why is it economic historian, Werner Sombart said, "The most gifted men have made the most fundamental mistakes predicting the economic future?"

Alan Greenspan and past chairman of the Federal Reserve Board, Arthur F. Burns (1970-78), see "inflation" as a major threat to the free enterprise system. Unsettling as it may be, from any historical and politico-economic-sociological point of view, both Karl Marx and Joseph Schumpeter, pursuing different lines of reasoning entirely to predict an eventual downfall of capitalism, disregard inflation completely! Neither needs inflation to explain capitalism's weaknesses. Certainly there is nobody in the US Congress with knowledge of macroeconomics that thinks even for a day the United States has it made. Our economic stability depends upon how much confidence we have in the future.

Those among us who have always had economic security cannot really be blamed as they simply brush off Karl Marx as; oh, that guy; well, he was just wrong. Harvard's economic professor during the nineteen thirties Joseph Schumpeter, however, is most famous for "espousing the entrepreneur as the dynamic factor fostering the business cycle." How then can Schumpeter arrive at the same final conclusion as Marx? Why is it one time famous Rutgers economics professor Arthur F. Burns doesn't disregard the thinking process of either Marx or Schumpeter? Schumpeter's book, "Capitalism, Socialism and Democracy," points out how the very efficient machinery of capitalism can leave many good people behind. Even the ambitious and well-meaning may be injured or become ill. The well motivated get depressed and develop anxieties. Seemingly ideal marriages end in bitter divorce. One spouse or both may fall prey to alcohol or some other "escape." Incentives provide the best way to get the job done, but, as Schumpeter clearly states, "Capitalism cannot survive without well thought out socialism."

Capitalism in America is surviving well, we hope. Those in power with hindsight and foresight should remember British economic scholar John Maynard Keynes who was well respected by former president Nixon. Historically it is documented Keynes espoused a departure from laissez-faire beginning in the nineteen twenties. Monopolistic practices, however, are still commonplace. Historically the Astors, father and son, reportedly owned one-fifth of America's wealth! Bill Gates perhaps has one thousandth of America's wealth or "whatever." Who cares really and so what? Well, some of his competitors care! It's a question of what's best for America in terms of global relationships. I remember seeing a Microsoft office in Glasgow, Scotland. Monopoly versus fair competition, what's best for 2003? What do you think?

Knowledge, however, is more important than money, or, as the Spanish saying goes: mas vale saber que haber" which means: "better to be wise than rich." Education is everything but what good is being educated if those around you are uneducated? The educated person becomes very frustrated. We do have forms of socialism in America. There's a world wide socialized system granting loans to protect our interests. The international monetary fund (IMF) serves to assist countries inter-related globally. A loan may be just enough to make it possible for a particular country to keep paying interest on the loan(s) it already has. No way out for that country till some Nobel prize winning economist shows those who govern the country how best to go about creating profitable export-import practices. Chili now progresses along quite well as a result. Argentina must do the same. Wonderful people in Argentina by the way from my brief experience.. Brazil shows a lot of how-to-do-it if we disregard its' sordid side. Brazil, the world's eighth largest economy, thanks heaven everyone in the world loves coffee!

In the US if you are one of the "working poor" (can't afford high cost insurance and do not own property), making ends meet and working regularly, should a devastating illness occur you can be treated as a "write off." However, nobody to my knowledge is motivated to be a write-off. Of course it's better to be insured. But, as already pointed out, what if your plan for medical coverage with premiums all paid up is suddenly bankrupted because of payments for staggering cost of other members' medical and surgical care? Other members of "your" plan incur such expense there's nothing left in the insurance pool should "you" need it, then what? Suddenly hospitalized you and your physician get the news your medical insurance plan, all paid-up, is "bankrupt!" The reason it comes as such a surprise the bankruptcy takes place abruptly. In other words checks in the millions of dollars to others in need of payments for medical-surgical services totally and suddenly depletes the reserves of the plan as it pertains to you!

Having spoken to a number of Canadian physicians about their "single payer plan" with the simple standard form, predictable payment in two weeks directly or reimbursing the patient, they love it! Of course they loved it more 20 years ago when a dollar Canadian was almost equal to a US dollar as opposed to currently about 65 cents! There are complaints Canadian physicians are not making quite enough in 2003. However, if a Canadian physician, by reputation, gets five cases to his competitor's one case he's financially five times better off! The management of organized medicine in cahoots with insurance lobbyists is negative about a Canadian Plan. Why though you wonder when so many US solo physicians tell of their willingness to serve patients for considerably less money if some sort of reasonable payment could be gotten "without all the hassle!" More sinful yet, solo physicians in the US who succumb financially as a result of injustices within such a complex "system," become even more miserable working for HMO's. Not only are they then paid less than most deserve, for patient evaluations and procedures, they are no longer able to continue their "style of practice." They must accept time limits with patients and must prescribe only what's available within the budgeted maintenance plan. Such a situation may translate into pure agony for the practicing doctor! This begs the question, "Do you think it's in your best interest as a patient to be evaluated by a doctor in anguish?"

Getting back to capitalism, whether it pertains to medical care or not, Joseph Schumpeter predicts it will be likely be destroyed out of its own inner processes. Schumpeter writes, "The spirit of the entrepreneur becomes damp as corporations become too large, too bureaucratic and impersonal. As affluence increases, thus providing expansion of social programs, this leads logically to a growing role of government. What follows is hostility towards America's institutions and animosity towards free enterprise. Government officials respond by navigating for more power for themselves. The general public is without enough time with their job, home, children and getting to work to become educated on the complexities of economics! As a result they become too passive to support free enterprise. As entrepreneurial endeavors languish even those well-educated in economics are to discover what exactly caused capitalism to fail too difficult for them to comprehend." (This may well be the public reaction in Argentina that led to insurrection in December 2001, and oh by the way, I was in Buenos Aires with my gal, Phyllis, as we missed tear gas by about a mile. Hearsay in Buenos Aires many among the wealthy own property and bank their money in neighboring Uruguay. Fascinating, isn't it?)

Capitalism abounds, but let's face it, America is socialized to quite an extent. If Schumpeter's predictions seem to have merit wouldn't a more uniform system of medical-surgical care, working more efficiently for doctor and patient, constitute improvement over the discombobulated socialized care systems in place in the US today? For our future, wouldn't this be an improved strategy "to preserve efficient capitalism?"

Worldwide there is much agreement that "capitalism is necessary for progress." Isn't taking care of those who become ill in a more streamlined and willing fashion going to make everyone feel better regarding how capitalist business is managed.? For a fair minded capitalist a little more empathy for those among us who get ill improves on a justification for our "competitive attitude."

For those who are monopolistic perhaps they are so obsessed with their job they don't think about the importance of good medical care for everyone. Capitalists of such ilk are very much at odds with head of the European Union's Competition Commission, Mr. Mario Monti, the courtly Italian who welcomes competition but not "dominance!" I suppose Mr. Monte asked former CEO of General Electric, Jack Welch, "Tell me, who do you think you are anyway?"

In retrospect as the Industrial Revolution slowly evolved there was created a class of industrial workers that toiled under appalling conditions. As capitalism grew, demands on workers increased. Job misery was so great the only escape was to get drunk. The magnitude of change was between 1750 and 1850. Empathizing idealists came along like most famous Karl Marx and Friedrich Engels. Their book, "Communist Manifesto" published in 1848 described the economic complexities facing humanity, with hopefully a way for oppressed to eventually emerge from poverty and the misery of working so hard and long there was no time for play. "Marxism" reactively was hyped as synonymous with the downfall of capitalism, but "communism" per se was not the threat as perceived, because passage of time has shown, sociologically, it could not have been then because it isn't now. It's "the worry about failure of capitalism per se" that has remained the constant threat to America and why some of its policies that smack of injustice remain. Lack of education about the realities of economics has been one big problem for America, and the 21st century is not a time for us to join together in a standing ovation for stupidity.

Early during his political life Richard Nixon proves to be a "communist fighter if there ever was one." By 1972, as President Nixon, his favorite national security advisor Henry Kissinger, working with Chou en lai, arranges for Nixon to visit the People's Republic of China. Perhaps only Henry Kissinger knows the details of the interpersonal relationship between Chou en lai and Nixon, but something happens that inspires Nixon. "We in America need not be afraid of communism," Richard Nixon writes in one of his books years after resigning as president. During the 21st century it now appears China is rapidly embracing capitalism. It's of the utmost importance the United States preserves its position as the major capitalistic world power. America needs to work closely with all friendly nations abroad like Russia. The Soviets are suffering discombobulated horrific financial problems having made too sudden a radical "jump" in economic policy. Such adjustment to benefit their masses may logically take 20 years or more! Russia is a great country their mighty industrial complex demonstrating in the past equal ability to America. Great countries best stick together and work together.

Having spent 20 days in Hong Kong during 1999 including the 50th year celebration of October 1st of that year, it became clear the Chinese are hardly fearful of capitalism. In fact 1999 marked a time when almost half the gross domestic product of China was being produced right in Hong Kong! In other words the six million strong of Hong Kong provided nearly half of the "trillion plus of China's annual gross product for 1999," almost equal to the remaining half produced by a population of 1.3 billion on China's mainland geographically slightly larger than the United States! Since 1999 the mainland population has increased their production and sales by perhaps 40 or more percent per year! China's gross national product has gained by 2003 to perhaps a third of that of the United States (!), a third of 9.5 plus trillion annual GNP, sensational news for the productive minded of China! Chinese economists, however, have formed no illusion China will become "one super productive Hong Kong without accumulating entirely too much inventory!" The United States for 2003 has stocked too many automobiles, not too promising with deflation and a drop in purchasing power showing there are limits to everything.

Overseas it's noticed many Americans flaunt, seem smug and complain too much. Many Americans selfishly involved with themselves ignore Karl Marx. For anyone interested in economics and sociology, however, Marx wrote the following that no American in 2003 should exclude from their thinking: "As capitalism evolves, small businesses disappear. Production concentrating in fewer enterprises means concentration of wealth in fewer hands. As the middle class is trimmed down more and more folks are compelled to sell their labor, living from month to month lacking any means of production. Over time more and more people become dependent upon casual employment (are proletarized). Overproduction increases! Such coincides with a slowing of consumer demand. Depression(s) follow. (We don't want that!) Militancy intensifies. Instruments of capitalism are taken over via eminent domain. Socialism becomes a logical result. (The US in such a case becomes no longer competitive on a global scale.) It's simply a matter of time. (OK Karl, we've got the picture, and we'll keep what you wrote in mind!)

Those making policy within organized medicine with families well cared for; insulated from malpractice actions much more so than the majority of community physicians, and through insurance plans so well protected need to think more about practicing physicians. What if some among the big wig families were part of the 45 million Americans with no medical care coverage at all? Are politicians giving much thought to practicing solo physicians given such a rough time trying to get paid for their services? If practicing solo physicians are unable to collect on their billings how can they purchase medical coverage insurance for their families let alone life insurance, plus an essential malpractice policy? Must all physicians as of 2003 become "groupies" to survive? And are physicians of the future going to be able to think independently or become group automatons? Where exactly are we heading, and why?

Thanks to radiologists and those who agree with the focus on major money doctors no longer treat doctors and their families without charge beginning by the nineteen sixties.. Organized medicine knows it, accepts it, and supports this contradiction to the Oath of Hippocrates. Are they concerned? No! Are politicians concerned at all about doctors in practice? No, their concern is for themselves! Are those of an "Ivory Tower" who train medical students to become physicians concerned what happens when doctors to be face community practice? No, but there are exceptions. The focus is on salaries and grants and training more medical students yet finding ways of devoting more time to other things. Whether more physicians are really needed to fulfill community requirements is not an obvious concern. Higher management of medical centers concentrates nearly all its energy obtaining funds any way they can. By not reducing the size of medical school classes helps maintain the level of funding. Medical center management focuses on an institutional image hyping research that may have great value for the future but lacks applicable value for the sick at the present time. There is tremendous focus on the institutional prestige of Nobel Prizes that do not bear on the quality of how medicine is practiced. (The prestigious Nobel Prize is awarded for "original work" in research.)

What about this departure from important principles contained within the Hippocratic Oath? During especially the past 25 years physicians increasingly become hardened and discard good will. Physician's secretaries blatantly ask other physicians if they have insurance. Hospitals no longer house physicians or members of their families free of charge as they did in the nineteen-sixties. It's an anxious money oriented world and for money this includes the doctor who becomes a patient.

By the nineteen-eighties there are cases of hospitalized physicians sent or nearly sent to premature graves as fellow doctors "go on the attack for insurance money? Is it safer in recent years to be without insurance? Perhaps that is the case more often than it should be. It's interesting to note when physicians are treated under Medicare the "MD" is typically left off the billing form. This assures the billing secretary will not waste time to so much as "ask" if the treating physician desires to give a fellow physician a break. Where money is concerned communication about it becomes awkward. Is the public at large critical of physicians being treated by other physicians without charge? No! Most as of 2003 assume physicians are treated free! To their doctor they say, "You mean you had to pay for 'your care,' I can hardly believe it!" "Are you sure you're not kidding me, I thought physicians were treated for nothing?"

In these modern times, after going through medical school, internship and residency and practicing 40 years, the "old doctor" becomes just another mostly worn out target for making a buck. It pays to stay healthy if you can! Even department secretaries in medical teaching hospitals, I've been told, work on a commission dunning physicians for money thought owed even after more than enough has been paid. The rationale is sometimes said to be a need for extra money to be put into some pool of money for "medical student training," (actor-medical student interaction video rooms)! All this in spite of a demographic fact there are already too many physicians in the United States competing with one another as part of the nation's health delivery economic problems! This however is not why physicians "fight each other," because fighting among physicians went on long before there were too many physicians, particularly in certain areas of the United States. In fact a battle of egos would go on if there were just two doctors in the same small town. Add a few lawyers to the same town and the two doctors would probably spend a lot of time in court testifying against each other! What's so astounding is how many doctors survive group partnerships. It must be worse than bad marriages! (Thank God I managed as a solo from 1963 to 1998 and in spite of pleading I never testified against another physician only in defense of a physician. As a solo my patients felt they were getting the best care. For those few who didn't they hopefully were mistaken!")

There's also this "pledging of allegiance to a hospital or medical center" that makes doctors on staff look important and trustworthy to those in the community by their being on that staff! As a fact some physicians are not so terrific, fail to keep up and perhaps no longer care that progress has left them behind. Preserving the image of a community hospital comes at the expense of "preserving mediocrity." Ironically among insecure physicians who habitually order nearly all the tests the hospital offers is chosen the chief of staff! Usually the chief of staff is not picked from surgeons willing to perform surgery at every turn regardless the anesthesiologist "verbalizes the patient is a poor risk," because these surgeons are too busy bringing in the bulk of Medicare and private insurance money. It's a "business!" A certain doctor may not be as fantastic as people in the community think but he's the one who makes it possible for the hospital to "pay its obligations." Nowadays hospitals have obligations that must be met! Some physicians suddenly realize the paradox, "The dumber you are the more money you make!" Is there a solution to this? It depends upon which goals society desires to meet. Is it to be quantity and a gamble for big money, or quality and less of a "money thing?" Is it going to privatization and more privatization or federal management along the lines of a federally managed system?

The big question asked, "Why haven't physicians taken the high moral ground, gotten together, and done something to improve the status quo? The answer in part is simple! First physicians starting practice usually have little idea about money and hospital politics. As to money, in the good old days now gone forever, one typically finishes medical training a little in debt. In the nineteen fifties it may be one to four thousand dollars. Indebtedness of physicians today commonly comes to six figures! Indebtedness entering practice is from 25 to 100 fold of what it used to be in the nineteen fifties! Even if wealthy by inheritance "Medicare controls what you'll do" especially within the hospital. It's virtually impossible to perform services for nothing even if you are by inheritance a billionaire! The hospital loses peer review status if any funny business is discovered. Someone from outside the community loop enters to find out exactly what is going on! Physicians are much less in charge, any control eroding steadily over the past 20 years. For the doctor starting out it's "go with the tide," especially married with a family, or quit.

Physicians begin practice in debt with obligations of office or part of an office lease and at least one employee. They are vulnerable for scrutiny by local doctors entrenched. The "hospital 'executive committee' is the behind the scenes power-base." (Who are these people?) It quickly becomes an obvious case of "play the game, compromise or quit" and get into something else! Mavericks in the nineteen sixties may survive. There is no such possibility any more.

Individualism is gone. It's welcome to the parade! Come on fellows, get with the system, but what a "system?"

A hospital then may be likened to a cathedral. You have a high priest, a hierarchy and the choirboys. A physician as "the new kid on the block" gets more than "molested." He or she soon gives up his or her preferred beliefs or "ideals" and willingly goes along with "an image oriented commercialized program." The risk of not going along is being "excommunicated," or translating all this into financial terms "being gradually starved to death for lack of patients or lack of referrals should any physician be a specialist. As a consumer advocate it redefines inefficiency.

The Cosa Nostra (Mafia) shows a more reasonable attitude! At least it's easier to understand. You know what you are getting into and that it's essential that you cooperate. It's like enlisting in the armed forces absent military training and equipment. The "medical mafia" however lacks an efficient tactical approach for serving those in distress with disease as it becomes more centered on itself. The physician is fooled since "mafias" do perform a public service!" There's the newspaper mafia. There's an insurance mafia for certain! The medical mafia for sake of achieving best medical care continues to become more withdrawn or removed from what a medical profession is supposed to do. What is the real purpose of becoming a doctor anyway? What is it the public requests of a doctor? What is it the public simply expects of a doctor? Is there something unreasonable about such public expectations?

"Competing HMOs" have added to the craziness! The U.S. Congress continues to let things stand as they probably have access to good medical care. Facts, however, reveal it's not always the case. How does a congressman know? They don't know. If they think they know and the Internet is the answer they are not enlightened at all. And what of physicians as a governor, becoming state politicians, congressmen and senators? If such an elected physician does not constitute the most sociologically displaced official imaginable, I'm baffled to know who does.

Even back in those good old days I remember one physician psychiatrist as new kid on the block that I came to know very well. He opens a branch office in Newport Beach California about 1961. He's not welcome or "accepted." He's too well trained and too bright. Nobody wants this kind of competition. His office phone as a result fails to ring (once) over a period of 14 months! It's as if a boycott is done via the telephone line! One would logically think he's got an "unlisted phone number," which would be incredibly stupid! He doesn't and in fact he is listed in the white pages and the yellow pages! This sociological phenomenon is referred to as "local medical hospital politics." Many people say, "I just don't believe it." The "big fish in the pond, however, gets the word out you refer to him, and 'we' find out about it, 'we' will not refer to you!" For this type thing the Justice Department is not able to help out. Maybe it's a case of "going after the wrong crime bosses."

The Robert Wood Foundation campaigns to focus attention on improving the quality of medical care in America. It is encouraging to learn there are people involved and convinced there's room for improvement. Dr. Don Berwick who founded the so-called "Institute for Healthcare Improvement," cites via Cox news service writer Julia Malone on 5/9/01, "It's not with pleasure to learn physicians polled were in 95% agreement that medical errors occur. The physician poll reportedly rates medical care in the United States as mediocre, as it consumed nearly 15% of the nation's gross national product. Managed Care then succeeds in reducing the cost conceivably well below 14%, but increases not only the agony among practitioners, but also the "mediocrity." So, there you have the results of Dr. Berwick's investigation? By the way the coroner's term for some of those errors: "therapeutic misadventures."

For medical care to improve two steps seem vital: (1) get rid of malpractice litigation and put in place arbitration, (For wrongdoing you have your license suspended temporarily or permanently.) and (2) treat patients conscientiously then pay the physician right away by the acceptance of "capitation." For a doctor to be a "doctor," pride of craft must take precedence over big money. Doctors can be "actors" too but there's this exception: " nobody sells tickets to a serious game of "medical-biz" as opposed to "show-biz." If big money is the focused objective then try being a movie star or movie producer, or a basketball, football or baseball star! Remember it's another "steep pyramid system," and there is plenty of room at the bottom right at the base of that pyramid where the odds are you'll be.

Improvement in medical care of course begins with the selection of candidates who believe they would like to be physicians. Later the best tactic is to instruct medical students in a way well in advance so they can prepare for the rude awakening of hospital politics upon entering practice. Letters of recommendation from medical center professors can help a little, however, the student must be noticed in some way otherwise how can a teaching center professor write a meaningful recommendation for a particular student, intern or resident? Even with wonderful recommendations a physician must be eventually "accepted" in the chosen community. The ultimate goal for those already in practice is to evaluate the new man or woman objectively and not slip as happens to the level of a high school fraternity. The physician's wife also needs to understand the seriousness of her husband's profession, a quintessential requirement! Ideals may best be preserved via a single payer type of health plan whereby physicians are confidently paid for their services in a timely manner. As matters stand now no amount of talent or brains can help physicians do better. Under present political arrangements if a doctor looks happy then look out! Check his or her diplomas to be certain they're real!

America's discombobulated system of socialized care obviously shows a lack of economic foresight. For example, a six years old comes down with an extremely sore throat and can barely swallow. The thermometer indicates a temperature of 103.5 degrees. To support an office the pediatrician needs perhaps fifty dollars to see the child, do a throat swab and prescribe penicillin. A day later, however, the youngster seems a little better then continues to improve. Mom optimistically chances it! She saves fifty dollars she couldn't spare and so unbeknownst to mother, child, neighbors and relatives, a slight albeit definite risk is taken without penicillin! Streptococcal bacteria may survive long enough to release toxic products damaging the child's heart, specifically and most commonly the mitral valve. Beyond the risk of this six years old getting rheumatic fever with management expense sufficient to put mom on welfare roles lies then a further risk the child's heart valve may need replacing or repairing in the distant future, say between 2025 and 2040. This defers a cost which will surely be in the six-figure range to an adult who, as a child, had strep throat but didn't receive penicillin because his mother couldn't afford fifty dollars! An ounce of prevention is worth a pound of cure as the adage goes.

Overlooking all predictions made by Karl Marx as regards capitalism and Schumpeter for capitalism failing, is it true what political science professors have said, "America is a stroke of luck in civilization?" To digress nostalgically one must think how lucky the opportunity for our Louisiana Purchase, why Napoleon Bonaparte sold it to us. What about Lewis and Clark and Sacajawea, the teenage Indian girl that overcame language barriers, saved the explorer's records from the river currents, to make that exploration a peaceful smashing success against all odds! Think how fortunate to explore the Columbia River first! Think how the Western US could have become part of Russia but for Spain using Spanish missions for strategic resistance. Think next how Mexico became independent from Spain and then how California became part of the US. Wonder now about Mexico taking California back in years to come with a new California capitol in Santa Ana! Is it proper for America to provide subsidized care for citizens of Mexico when Mexico provides paid for medical care for its citizens? It's about money. Shouldn't our strategy be carefully examined? What's behind the current trend? Why is it permitted to worsen? What is the economic impact of reversing our strategy? Medical care and who pays is central to these issues.

On the positive side things are much better around America particularly when you review the writings of English philosopher Thomas Hobbes (1588-1679), what he had to say long before the United States was envisioned. Hobbes describes a bleak picture of life among humans as nasty, brutish and short. Obviously good emanates as free enterprise progresses, however much of this good was forced out as a result of our destructive civil war of the nineteenth century. Consider "The Battle of Gettysburg, " that left a record of stench from 40,000 soldiers killed with 16,000 more wounded as North and South engaged in openly exposed military tactics. As America engages in their horrific civil war the British built the world's first subway system in London!

Good still emanates but we fought for the freedom of others in the first and nearly lost our own freedom in World War II both in the first half of the 20th century. Instead of maintaining appreciation for what was accomplished to rid ourselves of all the "Hobbism in America," Hobbism remains with us up to 2003 and much of it can, by my observations, be tied to failure to make available to all US citizens medical care if, when and where, needed. What is wrong with that idea? Why can't America's insurance lobbyists see this as progress? Instead a struggle continues to keep trying to eliminate that innate selfishness that leads mankind too often to some injurious fate. Are we going to avoid world war III in the 21st century? How positive is your opinion about that as we determine to democratize small countries for our selfish ends?

How "free" is free enterprise supposed to be? One wonders, "Is Alan Greenspan influenced by Ayn Rand? The best known novels by this Russian-American writer are "The Fountainhead" (1943), and "Atlas Shrugged" (1957). For economists there are important points to consider in these writings. When physicians, however, allow self-interest to completely overshadow altruism they are not the kinds of doctors I'd want. On the other hand too great a regard for the sick that overwhelms wears down the best of physicians working with patients with devastating illness. If a physician's mistakes contribute to the loss of a patient there's no forgetting. There is no practical way to confess the error(s) either! Ask any lawyer. On the other hand if a physician predicts a great outcome when all seems lost and helps win a struggle against disease there is a sharing of that great feeling Jonas Salk experienced when he dared "make that jump from monkey to man." With great confidence and against conceivably all expert predictions of the time, Salk proceeds to create a 100% successful polio vaccine.

Many years ago a fellow physician named "George H." was very influenced by reading "Atlas Shrugged." Involved in "Goldwater for president" politics, he suddenly quit exclaiming, "It was like a circus!" George philosophized and argued vehemently against all social services supported by tax revenue! He even favored "private coinage of money!" A year passed. About 1965 George experienced a very personal event and was threatened with a major loss. He was called at his busy office and notified his wife was grief stricken! Patient appointments were postponed. An emergency was declared because their little boy was missing! Searching his home and the local neighborhood to absolutely no avail Dr. George finally caved in, threw Atlas Shrugged to the wind, and summoned both the police and the fire department. "Tax paid servants" arrived in record time. Very quickly it was discovered their little lad was keeping extremely quiet, hiding way behind a lot of clothing in a large closet. Tax dollars paid off! Once in a great while you come to appreciate it personally.

Long ago in the nineteen fifties the cost for a full term delivery and pre-natal care, free of complications, was $300. By the nineteen nineties with so many hospital "write-offs." costs have skyrocketed partly due to so many cases unable to pay for obstetric care. To compensate for such write-offs, charges for a non-complicated newborn delivery without postpartum complications of any kind, in-hospital stay just 24 hours, are now 10,000!

For a fellow from Turkey working seven days a week in a pizza parlor he confronted hospital's higher management with permission to use my name. His wife's 24hour simple delivery was reduced to $8000! In another similar instance a respected Laguna Beach house painter (17 years prior he was an accountant in Mexico City.), given permission to use my name became afraid and paid the $10,000! Having delivered exactly 50 babies during internship at Harbor General Hospital in Torrance California, without any problems whatsoever, it's sad to learn of such charges that go along with other excesses and disappointments associated with "nineties medicine." Both new fathers had no medical insurance and paid the extravagant costs out of pocket! Even midwives jacked up their fees some 20 fold from the reasonable 100 dollar charge offered in Oregon in the early nineteen eighties. ($25 more for the pediatrician to visit the motel.)

For medical care like public health measures it is not a great idea to allow the free market to determine costs when you become seriously ill and unable to work. For the benefit of all it's essential to provide safe food and water and a safe hospital environment as well. There is properly a fiduciary responsibility to minimize risk of diagnostic procedures and treatments and provide safe prescriptions for patients in need. Isn't it amazing we enter now the 21st century with such obviousness to patients as well as their insurers more money for medical care is being shelled out for less and less?

Almost always there's the subjective judgment call to pick the right physician for a certain illness or injury. All too often a patient doesn't know which way to turn. The generalist must be depended upon to refer cases appropriately and not hang on to cases beyond their expertise. Regardless of who provides service for illness it cannot be done respectfully based on the same free market that provides paint to some construction project. The interpersonal relationship between physician and patient means a great deal. Patients are sensitive. They appreciate empathy from a physician provided it isn't overdone. And they appreciate financial consideration except when their insurance carrier pays exorbitantly, then nobody seems concerned..

Slightly more than two hundred years ago Edward Jenner, a British physician, made astute observations milk maids with "cow pox" were not susceptible to the worst scourge of mankind, namely variola or "small pox." This led to vaccination and successful cross over protection with eradication of the disease. The last known case of small pox occurred in Somalia in 1977, unless one counts two cases due to exposure in a laboratory in England in 1978. Historical accounts revealed Dr. Jenner was dressed down and nearly came to blows over his observations and proposals to "vaccinate." Economically the administration of his successful experiment didn't cost a trifle compared to the benefit to mankind that defies calculation. Interestingly "the US Canadian border was to great extent established by small pox. The virus was "an early example of germ warfare;" another reason to be thankful Edward Jenner found the way to get rid of it!

Small pox or variola comes in two viral forms impossible to distinguish in terms of molecular biology. Variola "major" causes a mortality rate of 25%. Variola "minor," also known as "alastrim," causes a mortality rate of 1%. Unable to be sure monkey pox, or cow pox, couldn't undergo genetic variation to virulence for humans, or that an unrecognized focus could emerge, or that biological warfare could reintroduce the virus, it is stored in four separate laboratories under very stringent controls. The world health organization (WHO) provides this means resulting in destruction of the remainder of the stocks worldwide. Vaccination is now mandatory for soldiers heading for a likely conflict in the Middle East sadly with fear of variola being used in germ warfare.

For capitalism and free enterprise to endure America's social systems should be more reasonably directed. Why not one medically oriented plan instead of the hodgepodge of managed plans like Medicare and Medicaid? (America now develops "one agency" for homeland security!) Why not try to improve on such publicized proceedings where judges, juries and lawyers determine etiology, treatment and compensation? A significant example "legally" incriminates silicone, injected directly or even within implants causing a host of symptoms, when through fundamental logic of medicine and chemistry and immunology it certainly never did? Silicone is oxygenated silicon. Silicon forms 28% of the earth's crust. Oxygen forms 47% of the earth's crust. Does oxygen cause weird symptoms? Does the human immune system make antibody to oxygen, or do tissue macrophages protect you from oxygen? Isn't oxygen good for you?

If a jury, with heads made of "tin," is persuaded to believe something that in fact isn't true it has a terrific psychological impact when such a verdict becomes well publicized. Next of all things a significant number of physicians begin to believe the jury's verdict, as though their verdict did actually establish a fact! Basic science taught in premedical and medical school is left in the van. Nobody thinks, including a lot of doctors. This shouldn't be. Why study chemistry?

Historically, in the nineteen sixties plastic surgeons met in Turkey for a conference when and where it was mentioned "silicone was going to become a 'legal target,' and plastic surgeons better take heed." Asbestos "dust," long known to cause asbestosis especially in heavy cigarette smokers exposed to asbestos dust for long periods has incited a rare neoplasm. It affects the lining of the lungs (or peritoneum) and has been named "mesotheleoma." Asbestos, dust or in solid form, remains a "legal target" with some substance perhaps but one wonders about the amount of validity of class action cases. Then, instead of leaving asbestos on pipes and other places alone, commissions are formed and workers suit up and receive orders to tear into schools raising all kinds of "dust," the very thing that's undesirable! Lead follows as another legal target as part of modern America's "courtroom schizophrenia." Lead poisoning is a well-studied subject. Toxic levels in the serum are 1.3mg per liter, carefully established decades ago. Of course committees meet and may agree to change the toxic mg per liter serum level to "homeopathic amounts." This seems necessary to help get legal cases going! As an occupational disease scores of general painters and boat builders, boat and bridge painters, workers exposed to cauldrons of hot lead for dipping galvanized fastenings over decades never got lead poisoning! These fellows never experienced so much as a wrist drop! Kids munching on chips of lead paint from cribs are prone acutely and rarely to a disorder of the brain associated with many symptoms and signs that are obvious and totally incapacitating. If your youngster is having a problem reading in the fourth grade, and that's it, get a tutor and spend some time with the young student but don't think that the difficulty reading is due to lead poisoning!

Lawyers have created many years of agony not only through what's perceived as medical malpractice but in other areas such as representing one widow harassing another widow and visa versa. One case both husbands were killed in a private airplane crash with nobody able to really determine the cause. Nobody knew if the crash was preventable and will never know. One such agonizing case began in the nineteen eighties when former US Navy neurosurgeon Fred Jackson, a friend of mine, crashed his Aero Commander aircraft into a hanger in Yucca Valley California. The lawsuit went on for years. Fred is remembered for "his 'take charge dynamic personality," also for the Jackson-Pratt valve utilized in cerebral spinal fluid shunts. It was invigorating to the point of fun to go on rounds with him, my last visit in Fallbrook California when he had just returned from Washington DC having played hand ball (or squash) with chief of staff, Admiral Zumwalt. Fred is missed. Lawsuits of "deep pocket" and "wrongful death" type are just too common the past 15 years. If abandoned, they won't be missed! Many lawyers agree.

Patent attorneys continue to go overboard for drug companies working the courtrooms for patents on ever so slightly redesigned drugs, touted then as new and improved, when there's no significant improvement at all. Newspaper reports tell of "patent estates that serve as legal minefields for competitors." These legal tactics discourage competition. Generic drugs are kept away from the public. Patients lured by free samples offered by their doctor wind up feeling a need to spend as much as thirty fold more for the patented trade rather than a generic. As a result they are unable to afford a good car, pay off their credit cards or even pay for proper food (nutrients). Kaiser-Permanente wisely uses time proven medications and generics. Oddly enough in the cholesterol lowering category it is said only 30% of patients biting the hook on such programs stay with it for more than one year. What good is that going to do? Why stay with it and then wind up broke and unable to afford good nutrition? How beneficial is that?

What is the sense of some "omnibus budget act," whereby a Medicare payment system awards a physician $7.90 instead of 80% of $48 for a follow up evaluation? It seems this ploy constituted a financial penalty for having patients seen in follow up too soon! Who decides when a patient is to be seen in follow up and the reason for making it two weeks or eight weeks? Is it the physician or someone in a building far away knowing nothing of the doctor patient relationship that for instance necessitates a follow up in three weeks instead of six? Why don't insurance carriers, especially those that manage Medicare, make a special effort to determine what billings are suspect of fraud, versus billings perfectly reasonable. Why not a quick phone call to the physician's office to clarify the reasoning as stated in the patient's chart? Isn't it a fact billions of dollars are paid out as a result of fraud schemes involving oxygen equipment, wheelchairs, crutches and various other equipment for home care? Why selectively punish physicians financially without any sensible reasoning for doing so? Why isn't practicing medicine "normal" anymore? Is the nightmare due to computers and people programming computers?

Sloppily managed systems involving disability and compensation cases all too often drag on to create much worry, fear, anxiety and depression. Legal firms handle hundreds of claims in a very impersonal statistical manner. Both diagnosis and treatment may be totally erroneous. A condition "carpal tunnel syndrome" may result in a payment for the doctor, and compensation for disability, when the patient's median nerve at the flexor portion of the wrist was never swollen, inflamed or squeezed at all! What is on the computer as carpal tunnel syndrome may be far from the truth but who is going to know this?

For capitalism and free enterprise to survive in America and for the entrepreneur to maintain enthusiasm an amount of necessary socialism, according to Joseph Schumpeter, must be well thought out. He refers to socialism that makes sense. He's not mentioning "socialized yachting," whereby every family is entitled to a sailboat or motor yacht, or, physical fitness socialism where all workouts in specified gymnasiums are paid for by the government. With the milk industry socialized and some families put on easy street with subsidies, still, nutritionally milk 'is' very important and therefore there is some justification. "Socialized coffee houses" where people come in, chat, build interpersonal relationships, and drink coffee all paid for would be wonderful for Brazil. A banker tells me coffee, after oil, is the number two export-import commodity in the world! For good medical care you really do not need a great deal of socialism but you do need capitation.

A civilized country must concentrate on "needs." It must be meticulous and lay out plans for the unfortunate sick. If nobody ever thinks, then errors on computers are not likely to ever be corrected! Physicians and patients as well as those who organize social plans must "think," not a good argument for computerizing physician's offices! Reflecting on 35 consecutive years of solo practice "each patient receiving the best of my thinking ability," it's not perfection but it's surely better than a computerized system that's nothing more than an extension of the "slide rule." It's personality and salesmanship that brings out the best and most helpful medical histories. Computer systems while absolutely necessary for banking, inventories, keeping track of the stock market and many other things, within the medical care setting also serve as an invitation for fraud as well as an invasion of privacy.

In America today fee for service medicine reasonably necessitates payment up front. Otherwise a "laborious game of collecting with all the various insurance carriers begins" thus creating distraction in offices short on collections. All too often when a patient's insurance finally pays, the payment for physician services goes directly to the patient! Overextended financially, or choosing to keep the money to pay for something else thought more urgent, the patient too often cashes the check and begins small "legal" monthly payments to the physician, or leaves town and pays nothing. Usually the physician gets paid over time, but why do carriers create this situation?

In the broad sweep of history "timing" is very important. For America it is a historical matter of immense importance especially when you learn exactly how 13 states of the union came to be 50 states! It's a good thing Carlos Juan Finlay, the Cuban physician of French and Scottish ancestry and the famous US public health service surgeon Walter Reed had not collaborated 100 years sooner proving "it was 'the mosquito' that transmitted yellow fever!" France's Napoleon Bonaparte able to contend with mosquitoes, within such an advantageous time frame, would not have sold us the Louisiana Purchase in 1803 whereby we got a million square miles of land for 15 million dollars! (2.5 cents an acre!) The Panama Canal would have been finished and owned by France a hundred years later!   Real estate wise, the mosquito helped America a great deal! World-wide however the mosquito transmitting malaria, one time killer of ten million yearly and once the prime killer of man, now kills only one tenth as many millions of persons per year, mostly children. Should some AIDs funds be used to assist those vulnerable to malaria?

Computer software pioneer Bill Gates has in place a philanthropic foundation that reaches the Chinese mainland helping China get rid of hepatitis B, a disease spread not so much by men having sex with men (MSM) but by the repetitious use of non sterile needles. A monumental philanthropic example, for America and the world, began in 1913 when US capitalist John D. Rockefeller established the Rockefeller Foundation dedicated to the welfare of mankind throughout the world! With son John Jr., by 1927, 183 million dollars was raised focusing much attention to yellow fever! By 1950 Max Theiler of Rockefeller's Division of Biology and Medicine was the recipient of the Nobel Prize for perfecting a safe 17D vaccine for yellow fever. Ten years before the Nobel Prize award Rockefeller Foundation gave 28 million doses of 17D vaccine free of charge to the health services of 33 countries as well as to our own US armed forces. (Will Bill Gates match the Rockefellers and choose to finance the best causes?)

Of great concern nowadays is money given to projects in the short run that fails to provide mankind with much in return. Pharmaceutical firms, while doing good things, concentrate on patents and profits. Research centers concentrate on whatever brings in "funding." "Gene knockout experiments in rodents," for example very popular by the nineteen nineties, become commonplace and nicely performed. Results are engaging. Now we have the human genome describing 35000 genes completed by private and government financed groups. Newspapers report this and people dream of "end runs," expecting results rather than promises for correcting human conditions that cannot be carried out. Employing antibody to block growth factor receptors on cancer cells sounds like a breakthrough. How significant is it? As to so much advice on how to live and eat, especially to keep coronary arteries from clogging, how come those tubes clog while most if not all of the other arterial channels remain wide open? How do diets and health tips allow that?

55 million dollars proved necessary along with a great deal of earned support to reward Stanley Prusiner, MD of the UCSF department of neurology the unshared 1997 Nobel Prize in medicine and physiology for his discovery of the "prion." Prusiner stayed with what he perceived correct for many years as almost everybody in sophisticated research "jumped ship." He discovered essentially a whole new way to come down with tragic brain disease heretofore unimagined. He

proved, by providing direct evidence, normal (prion) proteins could, in certain circumstances on their own, change form ("fold") and cascade into a pathologic (prion) isoform protein aggregate known as a form of amyloid. Prions folding into ordered amyloid aggregates, the brain has thus been transformed into a spongy sieve absent immune system responses and with no nucleic acids involved as the disease becomes "self-propagating!" Research for more details has been steadily continuing, involving "universal folding machines" called chaperones," and chimeras bridging species barriers. Dr. Prusiner has made the sociological transition of a researcher, without any friends, to one with so many friends at the present time he probably can't stand it. Human nature what it is there have been reports of jealous enemies out there forming "small groups of researchers still holding out for some "virus" to better explain all this," meaning you are really up against it trying to please everyone!

The incidence of "sporadic folded prion-protein disease" is one per million as opposed to one per hundred population with Alzheimer's disease, another kind of amyloid disease. (NEJM 2/20/03 pg.681) The prion folding into abnormality causes a human form of gray matter brain disease first described in the nineteen twenties by Creutzfeld and Jakob, brought into better focus by C. Miller Fisher in 1960. Another disease called Kuru, discovered in the fifties thought due to a "slow virus" (took a year to manifest), has been identified as a prion-protein-folding disease. Eliminating cannibalistic rituals like ceremonial rubbing of central nervous system remains over the skin and eating those remains, Kuru, identified in the jungle of New Guinea, was virtually eliminated. The adventuresome physician pediatrician of genius intellect, D, Carleton Gajdusek (Nobel laureate, medicine 1976) risked his life but for personal ability to develop successful relationships with cannibals of the Fore tribe. He was permitted to observe sacred ritual practices involving cannibals handling and eating dead remains without being put in a large kettle himself. A more recently identified human form of abnormal folding-prion-protein is known as "fatal familial insomnia." Reportedly less than 10% of folded prion cases have been due to the genetic mutation. Under 5% have been induced from medical and surgical treatment: patients who received cadaver sources of growth hormone (130 cases), dura mater transplants also from cadavers (110 cases), corneal transplants from cadavers (3 cases), neurosurgery (4 cases) and depth electrodes (2 cases).

"Mad sheep disease" due to abnormally folded prion-protein has been referred to as "scrapie," so named because those sheep progressively scrape against fence posts. "Mad cow disease," abnormal folded bovine prion-protein "spongioform encephalopathy," was traced and suspected transmitted by herds eating offal that included ground up sheep parts including diseased sheep brains. To support this a transmissible factor was managed transferred from one small experimental animal to another though transfer by eating per se remains speculative.

It's not certain eating beef or a hamburger from a mad steer or mad cow by itself caused the first recognized mini-epidemic of prion disease. This variant of Creutzfeld-Jacob disease occurred in young people (median age 26years), much earlier than the one per million sporadic cases aged 50 to 80 years. England experienced 127 variant cases, France (6 cases), Italy (1 case) Ireland (1 case), and Hong Kong (1 case). In England during 2000 there were 28 variant cases down to l7 in 2002 from a total of 127. The total of all variant cases has come to 139. The young variant Creutzfeld-Jakob folded prion-protein cases first identified in England in the nineteen nineties consisted of ten or so stricken by the disease in a cluster that understandably induced fear of a larger epidemic among the English population.

Eight billion dollars was spent destroying all suspected brain diseased cattle in England. The beef industry of the United Kingdom suffered a tragic economic setback as a result of "mad cow disease." There was widespread increasing concern and tough political decisions were made. The probability was you could have eaten a "mad cow burger" and not come down with anything, but psychologically "fear was instilled." More recently the familiar virus of hoof and mouth disease, that transmits only from animal to animal, created still another beef industry problem. Hopefully the beef industry in England has of now been reborn with healthy steers and cows being given unquestionably healthy feed. Meanwhile the psychological impact has still remained way out of proportion in terms of all possible worries people might have in terms of disease. In 1997 I had a steak in England.

While there's no mad cow threat in the United States there's always something to keep us on guard and cause anxiety. One example stems from the bewildering Minamata Bay disaster in Japan beginning in the nineteen fifties into the sixties. Methyl mercury ultimately is discovered spewing into Minamata bay from a company manufacturing polyvinyl chloride materials. Eating fish consuming such overwhelming amounts of this toxic form of mercury (Cerosan) causes toxic neurological disease in the form of blindness, inability to speak or balance properly in those of the Minamata area who fished and ate such fish regularly causing deaths as well. The unexpected social tragedy is very well remembered to this day.

A "mercury scare" not to eat swordfish and tuna hurt US industries greatly in the nineteen seventies. It all takes place before discovering fish tested positive for methyl-mercury in their meat neutralized or detoxified it with selenium, also present in the fish on a nearly perfect one to one basis, making the fish safe to eat! It is claimed ten thousand tons of toxic mercury is dumped into the ocean annually about half from volcanic eruptions. The ocean's fish continue to adapt, as have the harbor seals, and just recently I enjoyed a good swordfish dinner. (No sea lion meat on the menu.)

As for prevention and cure of diseases like Parkinson's disease or multiple sclerosis (MS), we seem at an impasse. In spite of huge sums of money spent via grants and generous gifts to support research, certainly in the US, maybe it's like "wrong way Corrigan," or not being smart enough, clever enough or lucky enough to arrive at a full understanding of these conditions.

Surely it wasn't easy for Edward Jenner, Ignaz Semmelweiss, Louis Pasteur, C.W. Long, William Morton, Joseph Lister, Carlos Finlay and others who made giant leaps for bettering medical care, but isn't it ironic so relatively little money was spent for such monumental advances? Money and lots of it that's the main focus of most everyone today has failed to bring happiness beyond that achieved being able to pay one's bills. Likewise money has not provided the sole means for us to get the answers we would like, to prevent, treat and cure so many identifiable illnesses. Some other ingredient has been sorely lacking, perhaps working more closely together and not worrying quite so much about who gets credit. (I believe I just stole that line from Harry Truman.)

And here's a message for all lawyers, nurses, hospital administrators and insurance executives and, as Walter Winchell used to say, "to all the ships at sea:" Over simplification is bad because things often aren't like they may seem. It calls to mind a surgeon who goes ahead and performs an operation on a patient who "wants" the surgery! The surgeon at the time is behind on his alimony payments and his ex wife's lawyer is trying to drive him crazy! Nurses are calling the surgeon "knife happy." The patient nevertheless begs the surgeon to go ahead and remove her gall bladder, although the gallstones were not bothering anything. She says, "If you don't operate, I'll probably never see my children again." Indeed her two children, now grown, admit they wouldn't visit their mother were she not hospitalized for surgery. The surgeon decides to perform the surgery and brings the family together. He gets rid of the gallstones along with a vestigial organ the lady didn't need and receives enough payment to catch up with his alimony. He accomplishes at least two social goods, if you consider paying your debts as one of them. Remember surgeons do save lives. Of course there is unnecessary surgery. The reasons for it become very complicated. Years ago listening attentively to a psychiatric history this nice lady tells me of her 38 surgical procedures! She must be "very, very family oriented!"

<u>CHAPTER II</u>

"HEALTH CARE - HOW DO WE FIX IT?"
&
The Seamy Side of Malpractice Politics

Since the late sixties all piecemeal attempts to address the financial burdens of health care had fallen short. Each state had its own agenda. Major medical teaching centers within each state were in competition for "federal funds." Their focus steadfastly remained on the task of "producing more physicians," paying little attention to how many were really needed countrywide, and in which locality all these new physicians would or could successfully practice. By the early nineteen eighties the skyrocketing cost of health delivery was at last seriously addressed. The big question was raised, "What are the people of America really getting for their health care dollars?" Were the masses getting a fair shake? Were even the wealthy and those in power receiving the "best care" based on wise judgment calls, or had expensive new technology seduced their physicians who in turn dazzled them like everyone else who became a patient. From the billions of dollars funded for research were there "enough applicable benefits trickling down?" Was it not a fact everybody, as part of the trend, was in some way being shortchanged?

With the threat of federal funds being reduced for research, teaching medical students and direct patient care, any number of schemes were devised within medical teaching centers to acquire other sources of funding, old and new. Maintaining employment of the Ph.D. in research, fearful of too many of them unemployed in the sixties was understandable. In the broad scheme of things, however, there were not so many successful financial tactics devised by "practicing physicians" in America's communities. "Solo doctors out in the trench" were feeling squeezed financially. At the same time the public was under the impression all practicing physicians were very rich.

The imposing economic disaster for the country nevertheless continued and by the nineteen nineties the budget for just the treatment of rheumatoid arthritis reportedly reached four billion dollars! Under "managed care," when medical care was officially declared "a business," the estimated financial cost for rheumatoid arthritis was reduced to just one billion dollars per year! For accountants working profit margins such news was wonderful. For physicians, however, and especially their patients, there was agony.

Unless one is convinced "the art of medical practice," or if you prefer "tender loving care" has no value whatever, in which case you might consider undergoing psychoanalysis, this largely federal financial burden, reduced, was accomplished by allowing increased misery among those suffering the pangs of rheumatoid disease. In addition it created more misery for those physicians exposed to rheumatoid cases trying their best to alleviate the symptoms and signs of this horrible disease. Was this supposed to be highly touted "nineties medicine," where those patients with deformed inflamed joints were simply to be told, "Here are the only pills we have available under our program so be sure and take them every day and good luck!" Granted by the year 2000 there were "those select well insured patients with proven rheumatoid arthritis," able to obtain one beneficial injection per month for $2000, "enough of a cost to buckle a person's knees, arthritis or no arthritis!"

Any long range plan to solve such dilemmas involves a major undertaking to start over, or, "simply turn over a new leaf," and step by step make things right. CAPITATION is essential! There is, however, a much shorter ranged plan that might cause some doctors, who have gotten rich, "peanut stand types or, in-hospital physicians who run cardio-pulmonary, pathological or radiological 'concessions'"), to squirm and become very anxious. On the other hand who knows (?), maybe not! They can just retire.

With so many American physicians presently discouraged, so many starting out deeply in debt and immediately systematized so to be unable to think for themselves, the president of the United States declares an "emergency" since to tell the truth there is one. He "militarizes all physicians and surgeons of the US!"

All employees of hospitals and medical teaching centers immediately come under the wing of the federal government. Living wills are reduced immediately by one third! Salaries for teaching staff are reduced 5%. Salaries for all employees of the nation's hospitals are reduced 5%. All equipment lease payments due from hospitals and medical centers are put on hold for 90 days. The federal government issues its first apologetic note to General Electric. In this note it is pointed out "GE" hasn't performed in the very best interest of the American public operating so much on "profit from credit" backing behind the scenes over fifty credit cards! In fact, in this regard they have been no better than post WW II credit dentists and car salesmen, like "Dr. Brady and Dr. Brumbach" and "Horse Trader Ed," all three one time of San Francisco. The note also states in view of completion of the human genome system with an understanding there are about 35000 genes that produce conceivably double that many enzyme systems GE's "images of parts inside the human body" have failed to solve too many mysterious problems. General Electric is asked to admit their commercial approach has been up to now pretty much of a flop, and they had best at least think about sticking with airplane engines and light bulbs. Furthermore the American public is growing tired of being instilled with "High Anxiety," (A recording of the song by Mel Brooks is included which refers to "fishing expeditions" carried out as a result of too much curiosity and entirely too much scanning.")

Rank for physicians could be quickly assigned, based on training and time in practice, instantly lowering the current drain on the nation's gross national product, at the same time establishing an excellent pay scale. A plan could be instituted whereby all educational training loan obligations are "written off," as an incentive for physicians to relocate from regions where too many exist to areas where perhaps no doctor is readily available at all. A well-trained heart surgeon, instead of waiting for years on the sidelines, might immediately put his or her developed skills to work. Why not get right to work to replace or repair heart valves, or perform a coronary endarterectomy for a patient who suffers with heart disease up north instead of waiting it out in southern California with good weather year 'round but extremely limited opportunity to apply oneself?

With a background of four years medical school, one year of internship, and five years of specialty residency and ten years in practice, the rank of "colonel" would be automatic. With four years residency, ten years in practice, "lieutenant colonel," three years residency, ten years in practice "major," two years, "captain," and so on.

Specifically, if a physician within such a federalized system were asked if willing to move, for instance from New York or Los Angeles to Georgia or Kansas, and the physician, regardless of rank agreed, there'd be no tricks. Buy "trick," this is defined in basic training when a drill sergeant asks, "How many of you new recruits can type, raise your hands." Ten raise their hands. "Good," now you "ten typists" start policing this area! If it can't be painted, pick it up!" Instead "doctors would be encouraged to be what they are supposed to be, 'doctors treating patients'."

Employing tactics of military type strategy for combating disease the MD under the new plan would be free, not assigned to any "base" or with need for a "gate pass." Incentives for placement in place the newly located physician is also offered an on-going education-plan to keep from falling behind. Identified wrongdoing becomes a signal for arbitration in the form of a hearing. Malpractice actions are of the past and the ultimate penalty for senseless negligence is loss of medical license. For patients within the newly located physician's area all visits are by mutual choice. Like purchasing an airline ticket, "You buy your ticket and you take your chances."

Under what we can now call "The Plan," along the lines of military science and tactics; in this case a war against suffering and disease in the United States, once the physician is located no further orders are issued. A top salary arbitrarily $300,000 per year ("colonel" and above) is put in place. The ranked physician is free to determine what patients need to be seen and to maintain a record of reasonably fulfilling a commitment to the community being served via keeping good patient records. Whether diagnostic tests are obtained is determined by the physician and not by the patient except in the case of hypochondriacs, and other kinds of patients, whereby the only means of successfully "treating" includes "a test to satisfy them." For patients who through perceived misunderstandings become a nuisance or threat to the physician, local law enforcement is quick to assist in every way.

If "The Plan" fails to meet a physician's liking then he or she has the freedom to quit at any time. Each quitter may seek alternatives such as selling surgical equipment to hospitals, playing the stock market, going into acting or into real estate, or proceeding on to ask the Department of Commerce for advice. There are a vast number of jobs available. You have to see the long list to believe it!

.

For those who were accepted to medical school out of the huge number of applicants and "major money," undisclosed at your interviews was the underlying motive, best advice is to drop out. Pursue a career to become a movie star like Michael Douglas or Jack Nicholas, or, Julia Roberts or Michele Pfeiffer. Better yet start practicing seriously with a basketball, football, or soccer ball. If you can learn "how to handle a ball, skillfully," and with huge crowds full of great expectations watching and opponents willing to knock your teeth out or pull your joints from their sockets, you will have that big opportunity to become rich. However, looking back at medical school being pretty tough, when you discover what it's like going back and forth, on some basketball court, football or soccer field in city after city you may yearn to return to that opportunity you had to finish medical school. You may ask if this brief big money period with risk of injury is worth it. You may realize too late the lasting value of a life long never ending "challenge" that constitutes the career of a physician and that it really is an honor to be selected to assume such a responsibility.

Should there not be enough T-men to protect the president if he initiated "The Plan," there are other ways of improving health care in America. To accomplish this, however, first and foremost, physicians, patients and the insurance companies must make some philosophical adjustments that may fall well short of fulfilling everyone's economic aspirations.

Having read about philosopher physician, Francois Rabelais (16th century), British philosopher and medical student, John Locke (17th century), and Swiss-French philosopher, Jean Jacques Rousseau (18th century), it seems agreeable to me that man is basically good. While we are unquestionably born into sin, all of us are what Locke called "blanks" at birth. Corruption occurs, so it seems to me, as we wittingly or unwittingly corrupt each other through interpersonal relationships as we advance in life developing goals. If then we eliminate, or weed out, that which corrupts by obviousness, it will automatically improve everyone's lives in general. This is logicical," isn't it?

At the top of the list where medical care is concerned is the problem of "money!" The concept of earning money so completely overshadows everything else, physicians and even very rich patients are blinded by a process that has backfired. Medical care can be excellent at the hugely expensive top of the pyramid. Further down, contrary to what you might be persuaded to think, medical care becomes excessive at the same time less than good and in some cases disgustingly poor even for the extremely wealthy. Cite the case of famed test pilot Howard Hughes! Even physicians since the eighties, unlike years before treated free of charge, are lured to snap at the bait only to wind up with excessive treatment within our present "system." This is made possible through fellow physicians fishing for business! Radiologists may well lead the pack in this mad race for "insurance money." Physicians nowadays unlike the sixties "do need insurance to cover themselves and their families should some "catastrophic illness strike." Procedures suggested and performed, however, often lack common sense not just medically but as pertains to economics. Physicians are in the same boat nowadays as all patients.

It's not just an emphasis on "scanners," whereby patients are evaluated "like pieces of airline luggage," but gradually over the past 20 years clinical medicine and good judgment has been replaced by "practicing molecular biology." This raises concern among physicians who intuitively know, even if they have failed to keep up, that we are not "in control of our DNA to RNA with translation into proteins." Remembered is the value of the stethoscope and ophthalmoscope taught to them years ago before the nation wide obsession to use gadgets and expensive machines every chance that comes along. They know too about fear instilled by persisting everyone, feeling fine or not, have numerous screening tests.

Destined to have an illness and die by age 50, is it good for you or your family to learn of this by age 40? Is it good for all concerned to live through treatments for eight consecutive years then die at 48, assets gone, nothing to leave your family some bank handling your hospital's financial policies making away with all or a large chunk of your accumulated assets? Unless you think this is "good," then "a major factor for fixing our present health delivery system is CAPITATION."

Keep in mind: a Ph.D. is not a physician, and neither a physician, patient, nor any pharmacist should be fooled. World around there is also quite a difference in the "attitude" conveyed among those with a Ph.D. Listening to a brilliant lecture by an organic chemist from Cambridge, England he conveys this obviousness he really enjoys his "chemistry!" The man enjoys what he is doing! It's wonderful fun for him. By contrast, chemists from America lecturing also about extremely interesting topics convey obviousness they also enjoy the floor of "that building they supervise." They show the audience their "special parking space." They exude a sense of being consumed with some fantasy that everyone in the entire world should be taking "the powerful tablet their group perfected," (granted, it was quite a feat!) and that all who take it will benefit. Keep in mind it is the physician who decides when why and who should take a medicine. Beware of getting caught up in this "factory to you concept."

Secondly on our list that corrupts hospital-physician-patient relationships is the THREAT OF MALPRACTICE. Experiences of the past 50 years reach presently a point where almost nobody trusts anyone! This becomes quite a negative sociological achievement if it's the goal of medical training to provide all citizens of the US the best medical care available commensurate with what can be taught up to the moment. Patients often expect too much. Some expect way too much! There are two fundamental reasons for this. The first reason patients have little or no knowledge of the "history of medical care." If you wait till you suddenly become ill, the history of medical care is hardly at that point in time an urgent consideration. The second reason involves that steady stream of highfalutin promises that all too often cannot be met and may not be met for 100 years (!), in concert with rapid advances in sophisticated technology.

At the very beginning of the 20th century, Harvey Cushing, for example is destined to become famous, and he began as a neurosurgeon at Johns Hopkins. (It was 1896.) William S. Halsted, America's most outstanding general surgeon, consoled Cushing for years there were so many failures! Have patients these days actually developed an opinion surgical care, as cited in this example, is a case of "see one, do one, teach one?" Has the public at large developed an opinion that all medical student graduates possess equal talent for developing such highly demanding skills?

Physicians on a break sitting in the hospital coffee shop listen on as this neurosurgeon exclaims, "A 'scan' is worth ten physical exams." It becomes perfectly clear the neurosurgeon is looking for something to do. Of course he is and he feels everyone in his area should have a MRI brain scan! Every surgeon lives to practice his or her trade. Certain patients also believe in "the magic of the knife." This combination of motivational factors leads to unnecessary surgery time and time again. This fact is in perfect accord with qualified critics evaluating this whole subject in retrospect quite objectively. There is, however, no escape from such peculiar situations. Of course subjecting any patient to unnecessary risks, whether it's drugs, anesthesia, major or even minor surgery provides a future basis for medical malpractice or negligence, or does it? Each interpersonal relationship, and how it develops, requires investigation of "all the factual details and then 'arbitration'." It is almost never a clear-cut set of circumstances ("almost").

After an l967 Hearing before members of the California legislature, presenting persuasive arguments for "no fault medical malpractice" legislation, came others from various walks of life asking for the very same thing. Ronald Reagan in the governor's office was subsequently bombarded by request after request. No-fault requests came from architects, engineers, and a variety of building contractors as well as sub contractors, they all get "no fault" should that law be passed for physicians. This was very disappointing, especially since I was the one presenting the arguments, three television stations recording, which took some nerve to say what I said. One John Allen of the Nettleship Company of Southern California persuaded Assemblyman Briggs ® Fullerton California, later a state senator ® to grill me. Assemblyman Briggs did a very good job, but I also answered every single thorny question exceedingly well. Becoming incensed with the grilling apparently both my eyes bulged! Since then, Briggs has spoken upon occasion of me as "fish eyes." Well it was a good try, however, no such law was enacted. It was about the time "no fault auto" passed in Massachusetts! Anything to do with automobiles and trucks constituted huge business, compared to medical malpractice that was, relatively speaking, "small business." Attorneys regardless suddenly got fearful they wouldn't have anything to do! Fair enough, they had to have a way to try to make a living.

There is a big difference, however, between a physician who makes a colossal mistake giving anti-coagulant therapy to a patient who is already bleeding, a common error, and an architect cooperating with budget squeezed developers resulting in a balcony or railing later giving way getting someone or two persons killed.

What about the 25 deaths or so each year in America from mislabeled blood? The worst scenario is giving type A blood to a type O recipient. It's a felony if done on purpose and the only legal plea is one of insanity. It most commonly is a result of a tragic accidental mix up and not necessarily negligence leading to a judgment of malpractice among investigated cases at least so far as I know.

Patients should realize all physicians make mistakes. The best physician is the one who discovers his own mistakes first. Lesser physicians have their mistakes discovered for them. The best patient is one who, in response to an essential need for an accurate medical history, gives an accurate and truthful account. The worst kind of patient is one who chooses to leave certain "essentials" out of the history that, unbeknownst, may be critical for accurate diagnosis. Very significant stressful factors omitted, something other than a correct interpretation may be entertained. If all this leads to unnecessary tests, then some unexpected terrible reaction to a medication that could otherwise have been avoided, who precisely is at fault? If a person faints in public and paramedics swoop in with no information whatever as to what led up to such an event, unnecessary diagnostics performed, unnecessary treatments administered, who's at fault? Paramedics are not doctors.

Is it fair following such circumstances for physicians to receive a threatening letter from a lawyer? Is it reasonable for a profession to have fellow physicians coming out of the woodwork to testify against you for the money and an "ego trip?" Is there doubt "money to be made often causes people to be willing to program themselves in a dishonest way?" Meanwhile is it fair to have a physician answering a " 244 question interrogatory," to cause a distraction from doing his or her best for other patients and upsetting the entire family? Is it fair to drag physicians through courtroom proceedings tiresome enough to wear out a judge, jury, and the physician, as the "practices of the 'law' are verbalized for days on end?" Is it fair, after somehow surviving such ravening rabble to proceed with another two years of appeals?

Is it fair for insurance carriers to learn of jury awards so out of touch with economic reality it staggers the imagination? Is it fair for the physician being sued, to receive a request from the carrier for an "admission of 'wrongdoing to go on record' to shorten the proceedings?" Is it fair to ask a physician for a guilty plea, when the requesting lawyers for the insurance carrier as well as the doctor know he or she is not "guilty" of anything? Is it better for society for such to go on, the efficiency of the process understood by just a few and not the public to "settle sooner" to avoid further proceedings" the sole purpose to settle, dollar-wise, for much less? Is it necessary for some to walk around with "mud on their badge displayed yet undeserved?" Why say guilty especially if you're not guilty to preserve the reservoir of insurance money?

Unlike the "death house doctor," the pathologist or radiologists who usually remain on the sidelines, there must not be a physician who ever practiced that didn't have a very bad day. In a very convoluted mix-up, likely never to be repeated, the best urologist I ever knew removed this terribly bad kidney to immediately discover it was the only kidney the patient had! Good God! All makeshift efforts employed, the patient died. Both patient and surgeon were victims. That the very ill patient didn't die slowly suffering total incapacitation associated with the frost of uremia did little to make the surgeon feel just fine. Decades later the surgeon hung on to the memory of that awful day, long after the deceased patient and his family or any of the relatives ceased to think about it anymore, unless of course someone brought it up.

A retired ear, nose and throat specialist from Pasadena California, so nice he must have been loved and missed by his patients, died so abruptly from a massive pulmonary embolus, it was as if he'd been shot in the chest with a ten gauge shot gun! The good doctor had just been transferred to one of the hospitals I attended. I looked forward to seeing him happy to evaluate his nervous system status for no charge. Just about five minutes after arriving to see him I was paged for a post-mortem examination! Afterwards, I telephoned the neurologist at the previous hospital asking, how, with such obvious deep leg vein thrombosis was it forgotten to request those very tight stockings? He said, with regret "So much was going on upon his admission, I simply forgot." I immediately wondered how many times I forgot and that perhaps my patients and I were just lucky.

Most physicians still in practice today have been taught this is something very simple that should always be done if the patient can not be ambulated to some degree. By not following this established procedure then technically this might constitute negligence! The real question that should be raised is whether this really does any good, whether this is truly preventative of pulmonary embolic disease. Specialists of the big city say the tight stockings simply don't work. That may indeed be the case. By today's standards, much more sophisticated prevention is indicated simply not available in outlying communities. How would a doctor feel practicing in a small town learning of this then being sued for not instituting some measure that, in reality, doesn't change an outcome anyway? Better watch out as you make inquiries traveling the "misinformation highway."

Now, 2003, the seamy side of medical care has been more and more revealed. Arbitration, however, should have long ago been put in place as a relief from the despicable and degrading "politics of medical mal-practice." It has grown like a "massive tree with its leafs shaped into "G," "R," "E's" and "D." At the root stage such growth was preventable if medical centers and hospitals displayed the wisdom and foresight to "back down with something as simple as an unexpected escalation of charges and over-charges so often perceived traumatically by so many patients. Of course once the tree was planted lawyers and insurance men were bound to water it so it would grow..

In order to understand why our medical or health delivery system in part has failed an analogy may help explain. The American Medical Association's political arm, beginning just a few years after WW II, "planted the seeds for this giant tree." Perhaps they were too dumb to know they were planting the beginnings of a what was to become a huge (fraudulent) oak." After all they were mostly sons of physicians who had watched their dads practice during the Great Depression. As sons of doctors they were not about to go through what most of their fathers experienced. With medicine having advanced by giant leaps, they decided they were going to go out and "make some real money on all those folk that were destined to get ill."

Wood technology, as an aside, is interesting. A tree is DNA, composed of mostly lignin and glucose polymers with cells that hold the critical amount of water to make the tree strong. The xylem brings the nutrients (sap) from the ground up to the branches that sprout the leaves. The xylem in a massive hardwood tree is quite complex, like the oak with four kinds of cells. Think about those trees as they talk to each other and to the two young boys in the recent movie, "Lord of the Ring (the twin towers)." It's worth a moment's thought.

My beginning example stemming from this obviously "fraudulent medical malpractice tree," has remained in my mind very well: Gladys Gresham versus "me" and the Regents of the University of California. It had its beginning in 1963, and went on for four years. The case was not amusing. It was senseless to someone outside the medical and legal profession. What was prosecuted was an "imagined event." What was prosecuted for four consecutive years never in truth happened! What was more even more fascinating, the prosecuting attorney "off the record," during my first deposition, admitted to the real facts (!), exclaiming both to me and my San Francisco barrister, Leighton Bledsoe, "I know, I know, but I'm anxious to get my 'eye teeth' into this type of legal matter." It seemed unbelievable, senseless and quite ridiculous.

Why didn't the regents of the University of California step in and quash the case? Why did UCSF consider their legal firm "defend" such a case? It was a matter of a medical bill that came to $2800, just too much for Gladys, or was it her insurance carrier, to pay? Furthermore, what was the purpose of pursuing this action against me the first four years of my private practice? Why was it allowed that I be personally "targeted?" As chief resident of neurology on the teaching service on the 7th floor of Moffitt Hospital the last six months of 1962 at UCSF, Gladys who I remember to this day was on my service and she, by virtue of her own behavior, unnecessarily prolonged her stay. Gladys "expected back surgery," but there was no reason for a surgeon to be summoned. There was reason for a psychiatrist, but you couldn't suggest that to Gladys! What did Glady's internist in Oregon, a member of the board of her medical insurance company, have to do with all this? What did he do to make himself look good in Gladys

Gresham's eyes? What was he put up to? Why was I to be the one to receive this "special treatment?" What did Gladys' doctor say to the Medford Oregon neurosurgeon to set things up so the neurosurgeon could testify against me? Those were good questions that made me wonder just what kind of a profession was the medical profession anyway besides taking care of patients?

Leighton Bledsoe, Esq. and I had never met until he picked me up at San Francisco airport in 1964. He was amazed then remembered I had been a very personal friend of his former legal partner, "a hell on wheels barrister, " Elliott 'Bud' Leighton." Bud was a bit too much for Leighton Bledsoe, understandably. We began with a few laughs and then Leighton talked philosophically and said, "Ted, I'll be honest, I've given up some ideals and have resolved to practice law, do what I am supposed to do, and try to "enjoy life." I was frankly stunned though about his comment "giving up ideals." I began to reflect on those days as a kid "going through the 'fun house' at the beach in San Francisco," and hearing "infectious laugh." Enjoying life for me was to explore what was going on "inside the medical-legal fun house of fraud." Sadder yet I had heard physicians saying they had given up their ideals. I wanted to understand all this if possible. Maybe it was better physicians never married! Regardless, I was not interested in giving up any "ideals." At any rate Leighton Bledsoe and I never became personal enemies, not at all. I hope he found happiness in his profession and that he enjoyed life as he tried to plan. I have certainly enjoyed mine, even though much was not in any way what I planned.

"Maybe I should have been a boxer," so said professor of neurology at UCSF, Donald Macrae. "Ah Ted," he said one day, "You should have been a boxer!" Never having spoken with boxer Mike Tyson I can relate and think about "why he bit Holyfield's ear" and "Lennox Lewis' leg." It was "an explosion of immense frustration," the likes of it only understood by big time boxers. "Life is like boxing," Cus D'Amato was quoted as saying and he was correct because life can be frustrating! Have a good laugh whenever you can!   Sometimes things get so crazy it's the only sensible thing to do.

During internship doctors are persuaded to take out a malpractice policy with Medical Protective Company of Indiana. It cost $20 a year in July 1958? There seems no need for the malpractice policy but for 20 bucks, why not? The "pitch," what if you want to give a pill to someone over your neighborhood fence, and instead of happiness there's an unhappy result? Who knows, I might do that some day if I know the person being a good hearted guy. Now I'm "insured." Do I read all the small print on the policy? Of course I don't. Who reads all the small print when you rent a car?

Why was a case with no substance whatsoever permitted to bother me during my first four years of solo private practice? Locating July 1963 at 318 North Newport Boulevard in Newport Beach as the first and only neurologist on that coastline and the first neurolgist on the staff of Hoag Presbyterian Hospital, why was I bothered with all this nonsense? What was wrong with the Regents of the University of California anyway? What was wrong with higher management at UCSF? Upon moving to Sacramento, as the second neurologist to ever practice there as a relief to neurologist Howard Petzhold who had not had a vacation in 14 years (!), why did Gresham v. "me and UC" continue on to a point of harassment? Why did Medical Protective Company that had upped my rate to $100 a year, automatically offer me no further coverage when I moved to Sacramento? What was that about? There was no other explanation except Gladys Gresham.

Richard M. Sangster, of the legal office of Bledsoe, Smith, Cathcart, Johnson and Rogers of San Francisco, sent via registered mail, a three page letter to me, dated September 8, 1967. In the letter he states "If I refused to cooperate I would be making a serious mistake which could result in substantial detriment to me, and a denial of protective insurance coverage by UCSF? The letter also stated the plaintiff, Gladys Gresham, was asking for a judgment of $600,000! case No. 535,566, now pending in the Superior Court for the City and County of San Francisco, is set for trial on September 25, 1967 at 9:30 a.m., in Dept. No. One on the fourth floor of the City Hall of the City and County of San Francisco. You are sued as an "individual defendant," in addition to the Regents of the University of California.

A few days earlier a lawyer from that firm telephoned me in Sacramento to frighten me into cooperating. I told that attorney on the phone no matter what had transpired I would not show up for the courtroom proceedings, unless I was paid for each day the equivalent of what patients were paying me at that time. He said I would be ruined for life as a practitioner in California? When, in fact, I kept my word and did not show up, what do you think happened? Make a guess! Have you guessed the outcome yet? Case No. 535,566 was at last settled on September 15,1967 for how much? Please make a guess, and jot the settlement figure down on a piece of paper before you read further.

That was not the end of it. A representative from Imperial insurance telephoned some months later to relate he had heard rumors circulated I was a terrible neurologist, and no one should have anything to do with me, whereupon he personally heard from patients I had treated quite the opposite opinion. I replied, with tongue in cheek, "not that I'm the 'Lord Blears' (referring to the wrestler) of neurology," but I was spoon fed and trained by Professor Donald Macrae at UCSF, who for all I know, could arguably be the finest clinical neurologist that ever lived. Even being dumb with that kind of personal instruction I would be competent!

Sociologically, it was pertinent to try and figure out the point of the rumor(s). From what was said it seemed obvious the idea was to prevent any patients from ever seeing me. This was a bum rap especially since I was born in San Francisco attended US Grant grammar school and my junior year of high school (Lowell) in San Francisco. After four years in the Security Service, nearly three years in Germany monitoring the whereabouts of Russian bombers and Mig 15's, attended UC Berkeley and UCSF, pretty much all expenses paid by "the California taxpayers!" One would think the taxpayers of California would be entitled to some reasonable return for those dollars. Were these nasty rumors started by someone from Nebraska, or Kansas? What's going on?

I completed a questionnaire sent January 28, 1963 regarding Gresham v U.C. During that period I was away from UCSF, 7th Floor spending my last six months of neurological residency at San Francisco General Hospital. The celebrated former neurosurgeon, turned neurologist and epileptologist, founder of the UCSF department Robert Burns Aird, retired his chairmanship of UCSF neurology Dec. 31, 1962. My claim to fame was being his last chief resident under his chairmanship. Bob Aird figured I was good for "something" otherwise why were we pals through life me the last physician to visit him, deaf but sharp as a tack, a few weeks before he died January 28th 2000 at the age of 96. I also attended his memorial service held at Mill Valley Memorial Church on March 11, 2000, along with Dr. Aird's two sons and daughter and Steve Hauser, MD, neuroscience scholar, and present chairman of the UCSF department of neurology. Bob Aird never knew about the Gresham case, never mentioned it to me, and I never mentioned it to him. We never engaged in stupid conversation.

Had Bob Aird been apprised of this matter would it have been prevented from becoming a major legal threat? Perhaps there was something going on to push this fraudulent action beyond the control of UCSF, its professors as well as the legal profession? Gladys Gresham "dreamt she had a second spinal tap and suffered harm" when in fact there was no "second" spinal tap that took place. It was made up. The record revealed one tap that went perfectly, no problems obtaining spinal fluid findings at all, and no problems obtaining a perfectly adequate x ray contrast study of her lower spinal column that she tolerated very well. Furthermore during my entire practicing life I never had to repeat my first and only spinal tap. In internship I occasionally helped other doctors with the procedure. A narrow gauge needle was always preferred to minimize the chance of a post spinal tap headache from cerebrospinal fluid leakage through a larger than necessary needle hole in the sac that holds the spinal "shock absorber" fluid. Charted notes said she was up the next morning cheerfully visiting her friend on the 11th floor! What the suit referred to never happened!

February 4, 1964 brought with it a letter this time from Medical Protective Co. of Fort Wayne Indiana (my "neighborhood fence policy of 1958"). They had assigned the Gresham case as No. 025232. Mr. R.E. Jensen asked my full cooperation to reassure Medical Protective the UCSF insurance policy coverage "fully protected me." Leighton Bledsoe, Esq. then wrote on May 6, 1964 about submitted interrogatories received from Gladys Gresham. Summarizing Gladys Gresham v. "me and the UC Regents, who probably knew nothing about it at this point, had gone forward with "fraudulent legal practices of the law" four consecutive years," asking for a settlement of $600,000!

The May 6, 1964 Leighton Bledsoe letter also stated their firm was in the dark about the basis for the Gresham action as much as I was. Gladys now claimed pains, limping, dragging of her lower limbs. Her attorney in Oregon "thought it all came from her myelogram at UCSF!" A Medford neurosurgeon performed a laminectomy on her "cervical spine," explaining to Gladys the procedure at UCSF should not have been done. A deposition from her Medford neurosurgeon was to be obtained and Gladys was to come to San Francisco for exams by both a neurosurgeon and orthopedist. Interrogatories were then to be sent to me in Newport Beach that should be returned for "editing" and sent back for my signature. Thereafter Gladys Gresham's lawyer was willing to fly to Newport Beach to obtain my testimony by deposition, with the Bledsoe firm to employ attorneys in southern California to represent me and importantly confer with me before my testimony is taken. Why were they pushing this fraudulent action so far? Why was the UCSF medical chart disregarded? It revealed no mention of a second spinal tap whatsoever by anyone?

In Newport Beach by virtue of still another totally unplanned action I had entered into a local political hornet's nest and "clashed head on with local henchmen of organized medicine."

Awareness of this conflict to be which was to reach Shakespearean proportions was by the mid-November 1964! From July 2, 1963, seeing my first patient in private neurological practice I had only four and one half months of being the happiest doctor in practice in the US. Innocent as a babe in the woods, or so I thought, the ax of medical hospital politics came down. What then ensued was intended to destroy a man's soul.

As the first and only neurologist on the staff at Hoag Memorial Hospital in Newport Beach and the only neurologist on the coast between Long Beach and San Diego I was the best! Furthermore my training at UCSF was so exceptional, even if dumb I would have been useful. Was it being haughty? There was no personal awareness of it. If I presented myself as too happy in medical practice and this ticked off some local politicians of medicine then my plea, your honor, is "guilty as charged." Except for a neurosurgeon who dropped out of his final year of residency to come to Newport at a critical time to satisfy the Hoag staff, nobody knew anything in detail about neurological diseases. It was difficult for physicians to know what kind of case was appropriate to refer to a neurologist rather than a neurosurgeon. After a couple of talks before the hospital staff, however, everything had begun to fall into place. I thought the staff was happy and the hospital was better off having a neurologist as well as a neurosurgeon. Instead it was planned I'd descend from top (the only) neurologist to "the duke of the doghouse, and soon!" Hospital politics made what I had heard about politics along the Potomac seem like child's play. God forbid (I imagined) if I got sick at Hoag and needed surgery. It crossed my mind they would carve me up, pickle my brain and float it in a jar for display in the pathology lab. "See that specimen up there!" "Where?" "There! (A doctor points to it)." "That's the intact brain of a physician that locked horns with the local reps of the American Medical Association!" I knew it was important to stay healthy facing the "double whammy" consisting of the Gresham aggravation and the local medical political situation.

Henry Hall MD, as chief of staff at Hoag at the time, hailed me one afternoon taking me for a short ride in his car. As we sat in the front seat he said members of the staff had asked him to talk to me. The reason: "I was making the staff look bad." He said when performing consultations, "I should write something that would make the referring doctor look good, at least better." (What was I supposed to say, I really wondered about this?) Dr. Hall strongly suggested, "I order more x rays and more 'tests' that the hospital offered." It was also strongly suggested I join the Orange County Medical Society located in Santa Ana. I replied, "That made no sense because as the only neurologist along the coast for a stretch of 100 miles I would not be able to see cases inland. There was no medical association on the coast. Driving to Santa Ana or Orange was a waste of time, and furthermore I do not like organized medical committees preferring just to meet with other doctors over a case when necessary.

Months passed and tensions increased. I set up Hoag Hospital's EMG facility, ordered and received their first EEG machine setting up a 16 bilateral lead system like Dr. Bill Garoutte taught at UCSF (Bill Garoutte was not just a genius but a very pleasant man and a great instructor especially of neurological anatomy). As a result there was Hoag's first EEG laboratory. In addition I trained three EEG technicians free of charge and got Hoag hospital national publicity from the myasthenia gravis society taking responsibility usually only undertaken at a major medical center. I liked Hoag and, in fact, still do! It has been a very good hospital. No general hospital has ever been able to claim perfection but Hoag's staff offered the statistical likelihood of getting a very good physician had you been hauled in having fallen out of some tree and I believe it remains so to 2003. I liked many of the doctors on the staff and still do. We got along until local hospital politics had to get in the way. Most of the staff seemed innocent of politics, just wanted to get along peacefully and cause no trouble. Seeing patients was enough of a challenge forgetting notions about having control of all doctors on the staff. To avoid trouble you nevertheless had to compromise, if not for yourself for your wife and children, in order to make a living.

"The local kingpin, Harry Stickler, MD, was from Nebraska." He was a nice fellow, also a good physician with a great feel for managing patients. He had been a pediatrician who left practice for more years of training to become a cardiologist. Dr. Stickler confronted me, however, in a more forceful philosophical manner than the chief of staff. This was more than just being some "new kid on the block" when, after hazing, you're at last accepted as you are. Harry Stickler was "the big fish in the pond. There was no question about it." He got me upset explaining the way things were going to be and that it was going to be that way no matter where I might go anywhere in the United States.

In response I intimidated him. I scared him but I didn't hit him. I didn't lay a hand or touch him in any way. Still he became so emotionally upset he was later taken to the emergency room with a severe asthmatic attack. A similar thing happened involved Mrs. Winifred Bacon, the hospital administrator. After the Stickler confrontation all I did was raise my voice with that certain lady asking what was going on (!). I banged my fist on her desktop! She and Stickler could have died in the ER and the medical profession would be better off without such people. I asked myself who in the hell do they think they are and how do some people get that way? Born in California and educated mostly on California taxpayer money "why" was such a physician prevented from giving back the taxpayers their money's worth? It wasn't going to be easy like you imagine if you're naïve. "Post asthmatically," word was put out if anyone on the staff referred any patient to me, doctors would not refer to them. Still it was possible to carry out what I was supposed to do for those patients evaluated and, according to physician Allen Cottle MD (USC), I got rid of all the epilepsy in the community within those three years in Newport Beach.

The failure seemed a result of not standing upon the hallowed ground and "pledging allegiance to brick and mortar or the hospital building itself." As tensions mounted publicity mounted. The ACLU in Los Angeles learned of the situation. The ACLU arranged for me to be flown all expenses paid to New York City being ushered then to Montifiore Hospital in the Bronx. Before the television camera of National Educational TV I described the situation of being "boycotted" naming names of the few physicians responsible who influenced almost the entire staff of Hoag Hospital. This 30minute "show," was immediately taken to Chicago. It was played before AMA big wig politicians. The idea was to generate a public airing by getting their response (there's always two sides to every story thus opening my position to criticism) to make the program an engaging educational telecast for 1hour on NETV. Well, the AMA bigwigs were reportedly flabbergasted and refused to make any comment! (Come again the "conspiracy of silence.") They turned down their opportunity to explain the importance of their political position, but why?

The principle NETV network executive wrote me they needed the other side of the story to make a "program" and since the AMA refused to comment I could draw my own conclusions. NETV was sorry and truly sorry for me. There was a hint I was "blacklisted by the political will of the AMA." Overlooked entirely was the fact this whole ridiculous flap constituted, "restraint of trade!" Regardless the National Labor Relations Board was unable to give any help. I wrote to Jerry Brown's father, governor Pat Brown of California. He wrote back he certainly sympathized very much with my situation but didn't know precisely what his office practically could do. Unlike "On the Waterfront" I was alone without potential backing. It would have been great to "sound the charge," except it seemed certain nobody would follow. Furthermore if anyone did offer backing where exactly were we going to charge off to anyway?

It got rougher. For the last 18 months of the boycott my secretary quit. I ran my office alone, everything from sweeping the floor to examining patients. To that end I'm indebted to this day particularly to Allen Cottle MD of USC for continuing a steady stream of referrals and taking such an interest in my situation. He had a huge practice and was able to ignore political intimidation. Allen Cottle exemplified what a physician was supposed to be by opposing wrongdoing. A physician in need was a friend indeed! Allen relocated for semi retirement in Arizona in the nineties. Indirectly we have kept in touch. Both of us have some great memories which eventually that's all any of us have and they best be good ones. We have more divorces than most and if you knew the details it becomes understandable!

I chose a path that was best at least for me. For no amount of money was I rightly or wrongly going to be some "society doctor." Having been a salesman on television with some experience on stage Glen King, famous radio personality from Oakland who once offered a 5year contract for television, the goal then to "outsell Arthur Godfrey for Lipton Tea," came to Newport Beach for the rescue. Glen was simply a wonderful guy, very much education oriented. (I still have a copy of a Play of his with a medical twist called "Trauma in 310.") Glen King had a great interest in the medical profession. Glen convinced Peter McCoy and Jane Dreyfus of the William Morris Agency to sign me for a play. Luck was on our side since Peter and Jane in turn persuaded one of the nations' best actresses to come to Los Angeles, namely Mary Tahmin of Manhattan. Mary had understudied Ann Bancroft who, with Henry Fonda, turned "Two For The Seesaw" from opening as a disappointment in Philadelphia into a New York City hit with a faster paced "Broadway version." Mary then directed Two For The Seesaw in several cities. With Glen and Mary's help I made it. Mary showed me exactly what to do and we did it for 31 performances at the 330 seat Warner Playhouse on La Cienega in Hollywood. The cast of the "Adam's Family" came to see us. Marjorie Love Bell, Jane Wyman's secretary and a friend of Mary's made a special trip. The Los Angeles Times gave a 1page story of why I chose to quit the practice of medicine. I told the reporter I was "love starved, and that was the truth!" Quitting medicine was a definite decision at that time. But after performing a week or so getting way past what was nearly an insurmountable hurdle to get in acting shape to do this tough play, it became "automatic." I would think in flashes about all that medical education during a performance! Mary said I was another Dana Andrews. It was nice of her to say that because Dana Andrews was a good actor! "Two for the Seesaw" was one tough play for the male role with audience sympathy favoring the dancer from the Bronx, just two characters on stage for a three hour plus show.

Seeing patients during the day in Newport, doing the show at night it didn't seem right to give up as a physician. In spite of getting beat up by medical politicians at Hoag, I still had a vague feeling of guilt that identified one as a "consumer advocate.". "Two For The SeeSaw" was over the last day of October 1965 and there was an offer to do another play though SeeSaw lost money! The Watts Riots hurt Orange County attendance. There was "Hello Dolly" in Los Angeles and the World Series of Baseball. There was substantial box office embezzlement tough to prove that goes to show production is a tough business. In another eight months I turned over my patients to a Dana Point psychiatrist with good knowledge of neurology. It was off to Sacramento in the summer of 1966.

I was relief for Howard Petzhold MD. He had been the only neurologist in Sacramento for 14 years. He was exhausted and in need of a 6week vacation in Greece. Howard got his vacation! I became the only physician in Sacramento who "did his hair with a blow dryer" (in private by the way in those days). Soon I persuaded Assemblyman John P. Quimby (D) Rialto to do his hair that way. John looked in the mirror and said, "I'm giving up Wild Root for votes!" I came to know Jackie Habacher in the front office for the governor, and gradually got friendly with many lawmakers, at the same time very busy as the second neurologist in Sacramento.

On September 18, 1967 the final letter from Richard M. Sangster of Bledsoe, Smith, Cathcart, Johnson and Rogers of San Francisco at my office in Sacramento re: Gresham v. the Regents of the University of California. "Dear Dr. Thompson: Your letter dated September 15, in reply to my letter of September 8, has been received. The case against you and the Regents of the University of California was settled on September 15, for $2000. This sum is considerably less than our estimated cost of defending the case in trial. We considered, and still consider, the case to be one of highly questionable liability. Since there will be no trial, you may ignore our request for your attendance at the trial and pretrial conference. I am truly sorry that this case was settled. Your adverse attitude toward our judicial system, lawyers, and insurance companies was a factor that caused us concern. We accepted your statement that you were not going to appear at the trial despite your obligation under the insurance policy to do so. Our opponent could have made a big issue out of your absence at the trial. Since we had received no reply from you to our letter of July 18, 1967, and as of September 15, no reply to our follow up letter of September 8, we assumed you intended to persist in your announced refusal to appear at the trial. When we had an opportunity to settle on September 15, for $2000. We felt constrained to accept it.

Melvin Belli, who became "king of torts," certainly was not the blame for delay, heckle and harass. His mission was to make physicians accountable for their actions. Physicians were rightly "accountable" for their actions and their style of practice. With a medical license, if a patient is maimed or killed the event needs to be honestly recorded, not swept under a rug! Nobody ever has benefited from mistakes covered up! Like the "black box" in some aircraft which crashes, everyone concerned about that accident derives a benefit either directly or indirectly, and psychologically, by discovery of exactly why and how and what happened.

Coroners uncover therapeutic misadventures. Insurance companies are apprised of such events. Within the profession it's important to have every detail documented. What constitutes progress and brings about improvement is making a supreme effort daily not to repeat mistakes and to learn from what you did wrong when you experience your unexpected surprise.

Medical malpractice politics began from within the medical profession, and the blame for the tragic mess belongs within the political arm of the American Medical Association. Ten to 15 years after WWII AMA politics turned the matter of negligence into a "protection racket or political power tool." It involved every state and county medical society and in recent years hospital management directly. It was not the legal profession at the roots of the matter. Publicized legal cases have threatened to ruin well functioning hospitals. A tragic sudden cardiac death associated with elective cosmetic surgery has threatened to shut down a hospital with hundreds of patients with more difficult problems doing fine. Judges have also commented they're happy to get home at night having listened to so much rubbish concerning doctors fighting each other! The insurance industry has maintained its focus on calculated risks. Americans have characteristically been "insurance oriented." For insurance of any kind to work the principle of insurance needed to be kept in mind so as many pay hopefully only a few, by actuarial calculations, will need money from the insurance pool to survive their misfortune.

Unfortunately physicians who ultimately achieve status wielding political power over the practicing doctors do not have the brains or good sense of an Orson Welles, Henry J. Kaiser or Melvin Belli. The doctors who want to stay on the main road don't get involved in medical society politics. Demands on those who desire to control physicians-in-practice call for butt kissers and those who love committee meetings. It calls for people from advantaged backgrounds. It calls for those aspiring for someone to agree with them. Groupies fit nicely together and there are those who enjoy achieving a position whereby they can look down upon others. There are selfish narcissistic types full of love of self and admiration who revel at any praise from members of "women's clubs." Some would not qualify as mountebanks selling snake oil from a wagon. At least mountebanks allay anxieties if their potion proves harmless. The goal of the political arm of the American Medical Association (AMA) seems one of "instilling anxiety" to make all physicians fearful and nervous. (Be alert to the physician or researcher that drops his or her first name in favor of a first initial. This can be a bad omen. Be sure to ask, "What 'is' your first name?" Evaluate the response carefully. Sometimes it's perfectly okay.)

One reason for the medical malpractice mess like the Gresham v. UC case has stemmed from policies instituted to implement the so-called AMA's "one generation plan." In California 1962, the osteopaths of California became MD's by virtue of legislation passed in Sacramento. Actually not all of California's 1200 or so osteopaths wanted to make such a transition happy with their shingle that read, "Osteopathic physician." There were many dissidents! How did the AMA and the CMA convince them? How was the transition accomplished to please the politically oriented MDs in California anguishing over people in practice with a title, "osteopath?" Members of the California Medical Association had complained to California legislators for years. Something had to be done to get rid of the DO so why not make them all MD's! Any DO that refused was intimidated and told he or she would likely be denied malpractice insurance.

Instead of accepting Melvin Belli's invitations Saturday mornings to visit with him in his office in downtown San Francisco and discuss how to make things better medically and legally the medical profession right away retreated. Stanford moved all its medical facilities out of San

Francisco 35 miles south to Palo Alto California. UCSF also withdrew and refused to debate malpractice issues. No politically oriented physician I ever knew expressed any desire "to get into the ring and fight for what they believed to be reasonable and right for doctors." Instead, just the opposite took place. "Medical malpractice was transformed into this power tool.Virtually all practicing physicians had no choice but to go along."

Higher management of organized medicine decided the "negligence threat" was ideal for overall better control of practicing physicians. At the county levels countrywide, medical society politicians were encouraged to develop "in bed arrangements with certain lawyers or legal firms, as well as those involved with the politics of insurance." Coroner determinations called therapeutic misadventures, becoming civil matters, through collusion could be settled for extremely small amounts of money." That was the AMA's idea of capitation. Special preferential arrangements were made. Those of a medical society's "in group," destined to control all the other practicing physicians were super protected from malpractice actions since no physician was likely to be found to testify against any one of them. All other physicians were vulnerable.

I got acquainted with Ben Reid, top post WWII California Medical Association (CMA) lobbyist in late 1966. I complained about things at a legislative Hearing chaired by Assemblywoman Yvonne Brathwaite. Ben Reid after the Hearing walked with me down the hall and said, "Ted, don't complain, isn't it better that the profession runs itself." Years later I joined Paul Brown as the top lobbyist for the CMA at lunch. Paul Brown, also not a physician but representing that special interest group said to me, "One malpractice suit, that's a warning. Two actions, you pack your bags and leave town." That was early in 1970. Paul's comments confirmed that the "malpractice power tool stood firm as a threat to all California physicians." In the early sixties as aforementioned, this power tool was tested successfully against the dissident osteopaths, namely, "Change your shingle to MD in 1962 or you will not be able to obtain a (needed) malpractice insurance policy! It worked!

How was the political arm of the AMA able to wield such power over the entire US population? It wasn't hard. After all, if you became ill, who was needed? The answer was a "good doctor." This reminded me of Orson Welles' movie filmed in Vienna Austria in 1949 with a different twist of course. It was titled, "The Third Man." The AMA said in effect to all would be patients, "We have the penicillin and you don't!"

The "One Generation Plan," as good a name for the political strategy of the American Medical Association as any, determined politics at the top would assume full control of all aspects of medical care. At the grass roots level physicians, especially anesthesiologists, were studying for law degrees. Well, anything that went wrong, the surgeon always pointed the finger to the "gas passer" never acknowledging the patient truly was too poor a candidate for surgery. It didn't matter an anesthesiologist's pre-op evaluation cautioned the surgeon. He had to give a go ahead otherwise he wouldn't be summoned to perform anesthesia again. There was money to be made! Hospitals were expanding with larger staffs, taking on more equipment, larger payrolls.

In medical centers medical students were fascinated to learn of a certain professor who testified in court. The professor enjoyed the focus of attention. There was good money for such prestigious testimony, and a medical center professor that said something disparagingly on the stand about what happened in a particular alleged negligence case, could predictably do a lot of harm to a community physician being sued. The idea of physicians testifying against physicians eventually became something of great regularity. The ruination of certain doctor's practices became appalling but never thought of as extraordinary. There was the "Nork case" that involved the Mercy catholic hospitals in Sacramento and then there was the "Miofski case" that involved Sutter (protestant) hospitals in Sacramento. Each case required fifty million dollars in eventual settlements and bankrupted the insurance carrier! I had evaluated cases neurologically for Nork. I had met Miofski, the anesthesiologist, and once even met his pretty wife. He had three children as I recall. Both multiple malpractice tragedies needed someone like Sigmund Freud to explain. There were more guilty parties than Nork and Miofski but those two were the targets.

Control of doctors was of the utmost importance to the AMA. Equally important was money! Medicare meant, "lots of money!" Though Edward R. Annis, president of the AMA, lobbied seriously to prevent Medicare from being enacted it passed easily. Prior to that I got a laugh from the Orange County Medical Association saying, "If fees were lowered 15 percent (in 1965 $40 paid for a night in hospital, and neurological consultation was $35, office, $40 in hospital) it might have such impact Medicare's passage could be forestalled! In retrospect it was naïve to make such a comment. Strange though that the right wing of Orange County shuddering over the word "communism" and verbally touting "Atlas Shrugged," couldn't wait to take advantage of Medicare (socialism) unaware that Medicare was socialism!

When Medicare was enacted in 1967 there was "socialized medicine." Up in Canada, the Canadian Plan was being formed. It was "a single payer plan" which meant whether the recipient of the service paid up front or not "payment for service was regularly received within two weeks!" The Canadians, however, adopted "capitation;" and kept medical practice competitive. The Canadian Plan had all the makings for competition among Canadian physicians. The ones with the better reputations acquired more cases. One ophthalmologist with a great reputation might be asked to do ten cataract cases compared to a competitor's one case thus allowing that ophthalmologist to become ten times richer. The guaranteed payment for all procedures for all physicians in all Canadian provinces was set at a specified amount. It could have been $200 or some figure too low to be accepted by "America's trained ophthalmologists" who was no better than a Canadian. The training was essentially equal.

It was the Canadian physician's "attitude" that was so appealing. The Canadians took a dim view of doctors getting rich at the expense of the sick. Becoming wealthy was perfectly okay, by inheritance, winning a lotto, real estate, or the stock market but not as a result of treating people in need of medicine or surgery. It was refreshing to be reminded of this first hand from physicians visiting London and Toronto at a Meeting in May 1981. The American way was significantly becoming more and more quite the opposite. It was, "Take advantage of the sick, financially, any way you can!" You wondered, "How did things get that way?"

US Congressman Henry A. Waxman (D) is well known. He is bright and I know he serves his constituency extremely well. Probably we disagree on many things, but that doesn't matter. I like him, and we were in touch not too long ago as I propose a change in the constitution (just a little change), however it seems to have no effect and I'm still waiting for the results. US

Congressman John E. Moss (D), representing his constituency over decades since the days of president Harry Truman is retired. He is well thought of as intelligent, considerate, and very thoughtful who I sincerely believe to be a tried and true worrier about the welfare of the American people, whom have I known personally since about 1970. Ralph Nader's "raiders" rated Congressman Moss, through his decades in congress as one of the ten best congressmen! Congressman Christopher Cox (R) of Newport Beach is another very intelligent ranking member of Congress who comes across very well, is an excellent speaker who gives credit where credit is due! You appreciate knowing him for his outstanding personality and that he represents his constituency very well. I like all three of these congressmen and have had contact with each to some degree having met Congressman Cox just a year or so ago. Of course these congressmen do not agree on many issues. It's good there's this disagreement! It gives the country balance! As a "lobbyist" you do not concern yourself with conservative or liberal but hope to maintain "balance," try to make democracy work in a country where most people are hard at work and simply don't know what is really going on except for ultimately death and taxes. Within corporate America corporate employees are pressed to understand what goes on within their own corporate "system." Translate all this and think about trying to change things in all fifty states and you realize it becomes a big problem! If you would like to make things better, just do the best you can, be as good as you can be, and, pay your taxes! If everyone does just that America can make it for centuries to come. Enjoy its comforts and all the good food for most, and hopefully 95% employment, and remind yourself to say a prayer for the future.

Years ago as assemblyman in the California legislature Henry Waxman and I were having friendly conversation at a Sacramento Medical Society meeting. On the subject of medical malpractice politics he pointed out a person in the group saying, "Ted, there's your problem." "Where?" "Over there!" He pointed to Dr. David Rubsamen who was then "the right hand medical malpractice man for the California Medical Association (CMA). David Rubsamen headed up the Journal of Malpractice, its articles enough to scare any practicing doctor even make his hair stand on end! I chose not to meet Dr. Rubsamen. Why meet someone you'd like to punch?

It took until Feb. 19, 1974 to pass on thoughts about malpractice politics in writing to then Assemblyman Waxman, chairman of the select committee on medical malpractice for California. Here were some of the points:

1. No perfect solution exists
2. Most sensible plan provides a climate for improving health delivery
3. Think of easily understood guidelines to avoid complications of a system,
4. Avoid State Comp like plan – Federal guidelines probably best.
5. Universal coverage!
6. End the secrecy of underwriting abuses
7. Limited reasonable claims with a catastrophic idea considered
8. Available inexpensive legal counsel
9. Powerful loss prevention mechanisms with open chart investigations.
10. Innovative techniques and incentives for preventing repetition of mistakes

Reasons for "No Fault" as the solution:

1. Present system benefits doctors and insurance men interested in a monopoly.
2. Only few lawyers and unrealistically successful plaintiffs benefit.
3. Existing malpractice claims and awards system inequitable
4. Millions of patients have lost confidence in their doctor with present system.
5. Malpractice publicity encourages people to seek care as litigants.
6. Physicians demoralized and indignant aware of weakness in the present system.
7. No fault replaces physician court testimony adverse to fellow physicians.
8. Helpful opinions further education rather than cover up ignorance.
9. It is not possible to weed out all imperfections of doctors, lawyers and insurance men.
10. To further medical education removal of malpractice threat would help.
11. Discovery, informed consent, and "res ipsa loquitur" create an on-going nightmare.
12. Economic, mental, and physical suffering accentuate an overall destructive policy.

On February 25, 1974 Assemblyman Waxman answers:

Dear Dr. Thompson:

I read with great interest your memorandum of February 19, 1974, in which you set forth your thoughts concerning no-fault malpractice insurance legislation.

I believe you have outlined a nearly exhaustive list of the advantages to society that would be offered through the institution of such a no-fault program. But, I was particularly impressed by your first point, namely, that no perfect solution exists to the multitude of problems associated with medical malpractice. Unfortunately, this applies to the present proposals for no-fault malpractice insurance. There are two major problems involved in setting up such a no-fault system; the first is to finding the "compensible event," that is, those instances in which compensation will be given in a no-fault system. The second is finding a means of financing such a system.

On the first issue, there have been several suggestions, none of which appear to be totally satisfactory. Perhaps the most feasible study on the subject was a survey of hospital records which is found in the appendix to the report of the Health Education and Welfare Secretary' Commission on Medical Malpractice. That study defined the compensible man as a disability caused by medical mismanagement. The term "medical mismanagement" includes both affirmative acts and negative acts, but does not imply that the management was necessarily improper. A number of hospital records were reviewed and it was determined that it was feasible to decide whether or not complications developed due to "medical mismanagement." On the other hand, a study conducted by Doctor David Rubsamen for the California Medical Association concluded that it is virtually impossible to define a compensible man under any no-fault system

Financing such a comprehensive no-fault system would present further problems, since it is likely that the number of claims would be extremely high. In short, careful study is needed to determine what the cost of such a system might eventually be.

The Committee is hopeful that further studies conducted on the subject of no-fault malpractice insurance will address these problems. Whereas you point out, the potential social advantages to no-fault insurance are indeed significant.

Finally let me thank you for taking the time and trouble to communicate your views on this important issue to me. I was please to meet you at the Sacramento Medical Society meeting.

Should you have any further comments or suggestions, please do not hesitate to pass   them along.

Sincerely,

Henry A. Waxman, Chairman Select
Committee on Medical Malpractice

Not brought out in this written communication with Assemblyman Waxman was the most important benefit of all from passage of no-fault medical malpractice legislation. This point was brought out as the primary reason for "no-fault" at the hearing before Assemblyman Briggs of Fullerton California, in 1967.

No-fault's most important benefit is that it discourages any "need to falsify medical files!" Unfortunately, and you can call it human nature and not be far off medical charts are not uncommonly redone to cover up something terrible that should not have happened!   The patient's "diagnosis may be changed for the record" so that the hospitalized person's medical record remains inaccurate until the chart is destroyed. However, the altered diagnosis obviously remains with the patient all his or her life!

The first instance of this brought to my attention was a chart changed entirely at Harbor General Hospital in Torrance, California in 1958. An infant was admitted with a fever. Spinal fluid examination was felt necessary to rule out nervous system involvement. The lady intern became nervous and extremely frustrated. Not just 1, but 28 (!) spinal taps were performed, mostly in the wrong places, and still no fluid for laboratory examination! The infant's spinal cord was damaged. The infant was discharged illness resolved with supportive care but with neurological damage, not fortunately to both lower limbs but just "one lower extremity." That person today has a medical record that was totally changed and has been told the disability was due to an infection in infancy. The disability, however, was due to an injury from a lumbar puncture needle. The lady intern was placed under psychiatric care. The last I was made aware she received psychotherapy and resumed practicing. Like many physicians her license should have been suspended at least for anything involving medical procedures. Perhaps she should have been encouraged to seek out some other occupation. There were very few women physicians in 1958 and that was presumably a consideration.

One can only guess how many thousands of medical charts have been revised in order to cover up surprising and unexpected undesirable events. 1980 was the year of the most recent chart revision brought to my attention in great detail. Upon discharge from hospital I followed the patient for months trying to provide some relief for his chronically painful post hospital experience. It was especially important because it involved a friend, Norman Nixon MD, professor of psychiatry at UC Irvine medical center, a fellow Rotarian and "patron of the arts in Orange County."

Arriving at South Coast hospital Laguna Beach California to do a consult during September 1980, I happened to pass the private room of a patient moaning, then heard a call, "Ted!" I entered the room to see Norman Nixon MD in agony! He had a swollen bluish right forearm and obviously heparin anticoagulant IV infiltration via the needle was the reason for his pain. I dashed out of the room to locate the floor nurse whom I knew very well because her young daughter had been a patient of mine for several years. She entered Dr. Nixon's room, alarmed at what she observed, quickly discontinued the infiltrated heparin IV. We then returned to the nurses' station and I reviewed Dr. Nixon's chart carefully from his admission a few days ago to the present. I returned to Dr Nixon's room consoling him and also aware he was in considerable pain.

The next day I went by to see my patient at the same time saying hello to Dr. Nixon. I also looked at Dr. Nixon's chart that revealed a totally different write up! The doctor's admission note was revised, all nurses' notes were revised, and there was no mention of what had transpired the night before! It was a different chart!

During examinations of Dr. Nixon's painful condition, at intervals in my office, he brought me a copy of his hospital record. It was of course the redone version. The original version no longer existed! He knew it and I knew it. There was no longer any charted evidence of what I came across that night discovering Dr. Nixon agonizing in pain. With the original chart no longer in existence, where was some of the evidence of all that had gone wrong? A "cover up" was a cover up, just the same as, in criminal court if you're "framed" you're framed! There were two shifts of nurses between my hospital visits but no personnel the second time I knew well enough to ask any thorny questions about Dr. Nixon, "particularly as an unofficial meddler!" The painful puffed up forearm that I witnessed "never happened?" I did note in "the new and improved hospital record," psychiatrist Nixon was seen by a hospital staff psychiatrist, John Burnham, MD. Impression was, "depressive reaction, resolving." More correctly it should have been "depressing hospital experience," and with luck the patient made it through anyway!

In other words it was not just a matter of the chart being partly falsified but part of "a hospital medical team management defense," to make a case of something psychologically wrong with Dr.Nixon. That ploy would further protect the hospital. "Isn't it a fact Dr. Nixon your swelled up, blue, painful forearm was imagined? Isn't it a fact, you, and your fellow physician friend, Dr. Thompson, conspired to invent a reason to bring an action against these fine doctors and this fine hospital?

What really topped off the whole experience about two months later I happened to be enjoying a piece of delicious pie in the doctor's dining room at South Coast Hospital, all alone except for our hospital chief administrator. He always seemed like a nice guy. Rambling on what a sensational job one "Charlene Vance" had done managing and preparing all the terrific food for patients and physicians at SCMC (the best really I've ever known anywhere in any hospital before or since), I politely said, "That was certainly a shame what happened to Dr. Nixon." He replied, "Dr. Nixon (!), say, he's quite 'paranoid,' isn't he?"

Dr. Nixon was a very intelligent mild mannered physician with no intention of suing any doctors or any hospital. The staff hurt him! He was injured by physician's orders. He was in a good deal of pain for many months! As a fellow physician, wasn't he permitted to even comment about his hospitalization misfortune? He wanted those responsible to realize what happened, and to play a role to help the staff avoid hurting someone else in the future in the same manner. It was so forward and simple! Nobody injured him intentionally! Everybody agreed with that. But, without "no-fault negligence," and an arbiter, the event had to be eliminated from the hospital's record to protect the hospital. Within such a litigious society, malpractice politics what they are, such fraudulent tactics have been understandable. Dr. Nixon never wished the hospital to shut down because part of the staff gave him an aching arm and shoulder. No wonder our society has gone backwards in so many respects! In respect to creating situations necessitating fraudulent activity we seem to be advancing, as a society, on fast forward.

Well Norman Nixon, MD passed away some years ago and much was philosophized between the two of us about what happened and how to deal with "what's done is done." It seemed tragic to me to see physicians treat another physician in this manner! In Dr. Nixon's case I sincerely think an admission of what happened and a heart felt apology would have relieved some of his pain. His suffering was "mental," I believe, along with the obvious physical components. He was so terribly disappointed in the attitude of the physicians and hospital staff. (By the way, even a hospitalized "lawyer" was to have no chance to sue successfully with "an altered hospital record!")

Herein is Norman Nixon's letter to the Board of South Coast Medical Center dated August 14, 1981. It's taken from my "confidential copy," in his file. Read it please and decide in your own mind if you think Dr. Nixon was "depressed." Do you think he was a grumpy old doctor that wanted to complain?

Dear Larry (Hunt), Chairman, and members of the Board:
South Coast Medical Center (SCMC), Laguna Beach, California

A recent 3-months' survey of patients hospitalized at Boston's Massachusetts General and Peter Bent Brigham hospitals concluded that 35 percent showed more pathology at discharge than was present when they were admitted. Errors of commission or omission made by doctors, nurses, technicians and/or other hospital personnel were primarily responsible.

Another study published in the New England Journal of Medicine concluded, that of 815 patients admitted, to Boston University Medical Center, during a 5month period, 290 (36 percent) suffered 500 medical mishaps. Some deaths were reported in both studies. A survey of patients admitted to SCMS probably would reveal comparable, even larger statistics.

I will try to summarize my unfortunate experience during hospitalization here from Thursday, 9/25/80, to Saturday, 10/10/80, for treatment of left leg phlebitis. Dr. Mark Johnston, my admitting physician, ordered a continuous intravenous infusion of a heparin solution (5000 units). This was started in one of the veins of my left hand, shortly after admission to the surgical ward. A McGaw pump with a warning bell was part of the IV set-up. The procedure seemed to go smoothly the first night, then the bell began sounding with increasing frequency on Friday and Saturday. A new McGaw pump was installed but the warning bell continued to ring sporadically and I became aware of what seemed to be leaking of the heparin solution at the needle site. However, members of the IV team (and ward nurses) kept assuring me all was well.

Reportedly, the 5member IV team is solely responsible for administering all IV fluids and medications on all wards, day and night. Sometimes, particularly during night shifts and on the weekend with the hospital staff shorthanded, the IV team member on duty did not respond for a long time. Occasionally several hours passed, after I reported to the ward nurse the warning bell was signaling trouble, and, I was experiencing discomfort at the needle site. Finally, late Saturday night (9/27), I insisted on calling the night superintendent of nurses, who responded promptly, withdrew the needle and restarted the heparin infusion in another vein in my left arm. No note of her action was recorded in the chart nor were most of the ministrations of the IV team, including the replacement of the McGaw pump.

By Monday morning (9/29) my left hand and forearm were swollen and inflamed due to heparin infiltration into the soft tissue of the hand. Soon, the entire left arm to shoulder, and much of my back was involved. Dr. Johnston removed the needle from the left, transferring the IV infusion to my right arm, and wrapped the injured arm with elastic bandage. There was little pain at that time, probably due to nerve damage. That same morning I reported to Dr. Johnston and the ward nurse that I had just experienced a sudden loss of hearing in my left ear, with loss of equilibrium and other vestibular symptoms. My hospital chart shows no record of this.

The pronounced edema, skin discoloration, etc; (my left arm was nearly twice normal size) subsided slowly after many weeks of treatment (physical therapy, ultrasound, packs, exercises by Mr. Monlux, medical supervision by Dr. Roper. The neuro-muscular symptoms have diminished, although I cannot type and many small muscle tasks are difficult. The numbness, tingling, and discomfort, in my left arm, hand to shoulder, continue, due to the residual damage to nerves and blood vessels. With no apparent change for months, the residual pathology probably will continue the rest of my life. The hearing loss (left) and loss of equilibrium are also unchanged. I was examined and tested by two ear specialists: Dr. Kent Combs, SCMC, and Dr. Howard House of Los Angeles; and by Dr. Ted Thompson, neurologist at SCMC. My general condition has improved however.

Heparin is a valuable, but potentially dangerous drug. When administered IV it reaches every part of the body almost instantly, necessitating careful monitoring day and night, Saturdays and Sundays included. When the limited services of the IV team are not available, other competent personnel, equally experienced, should be on duty to cover for them. Unfortunately, these guidelines were not followed in my case.

I can understand your concern regarding the continuing low patient census at SCMC. Adding a new professional building "to attract more physicians to South Laguna, and more patients to fill hospital beds," may help. Provided, of course that SCMC does not become part of the unwieldy medical-industrial complex, *and go far beyond the realistic health care needs of South Orange County.

Just as important, it seems to me, would be a concerted effort to improve our hospital's image so that more patients would choose SCMC, as their hospital of first choice, when hospitalization is necessary. As I sense the feeling in our community today, the former good image of "the hospital with a heart" has faded considerably. Much needs to be done to revive "Papa" Kroch's dream. Mishaps such as I experienced certainly do not help.

Sincerely,   *US News and World Report, August 17, 1981
                                              Medicine and Profits, Unhealthy Mixture p50

Norman Nixon, MD

Extract a little extra money from millions of persons and a tremendous profit can be made. Nobody is hurt too much. That seems to be the general attitude of corporate America. Directing attention to the pharmaceutical industry, is the skyrocketing cost of drugs due to greed or something else? Well, greed and the "middle man" (the distributors) are sure part of it, but, don't growl too much at the village pharmacist. If you want to do something to help the pharmaceutical industry lower consumer prices focus attention on "no-fault prescription malpractice." Tort law and negligence cases regarding drug reactions cause "the triple nightmare situation," one the drug companies, two the physicians who prescribe, and three the pharmacist. Such cases constitute the beau ideal keeping everyone paying big money for those malpractice policies. The awards can be large enough to bankrupt a small carrier. Small carriers can't afford top lobbyists to keep things from getting totally out of hand because that also takes a lot of money.

A 30fold increase over a generic may be your eventual cost for a trademark drug by virtue of being started on free samples by your "commercialized" physician. This can become altogether too much of a drain on your insurance plan or, for the vast majority of patients, ones' personal pocket book. Of course there is some sense to these high costs, even though a gut reaction indicates it makes no sense at all.

Part of the staggering cost is to defray the cost of television, periodical and newspaper advertising. Part of the high cost is to provide millions of dollars for legal firm representation that's divided, in order to simplify, into two general areas. The first is to provide millions of dollars for patent lawyers to "capitalize on the sluggishness of the current legal system." Their job is to prolong the monopolistic desire of the drug firm that holds the patent. They must hold off impending competition from other manufacturers anxious to be given "legal permission" to make the very same successful sales product" and sell it for a lot less. The second has to do with malpractice politics and the outlandish actions taken against the pharmaceutical industry.

One of my favorite dermatologists who I have known for decades, a gracious lady who would not intentionally hurt anybody, prescribed an antibiotic she had been using with luck and success for treatment of terribly disfiguring cases of acne. Such cases were responding quite satisfactorily. The short of it, a certain young man with acne also responded well to the prescription but, as chance would have it, he developed renal (kidney) side effects. The drug needed to be stopped immediately since it was the offending factor! Sometimes that ideal has not been carried out and there's nobody really to blame. Tragic side effects have occurred since therapeutics began and the greater number of patients who benefit equates with an increased chance for unwanted side effects.

The pharmaceutical firm got sued for manufacturing the drug. Never mind in certain medical situations the drug had been life saving. My dermatologist friend was sued of course upset since she wrote the prescription. Never mind she had other patients desperate to get rid of their acne that were doing just fine on this antibiotic. What really struck me the pharmacist got sued as well! All he did was take the proper antibiotic off his shelf, package it with proper directions as ordered by the physician, pick-up very few dollars profit handing the product to the patient or a member of the patient's family. Why was the pharmacist nailed? What was his wrongdoing? Why did a lawyer upset his life with aggravations, interrogatories, and investigations to then be insisted upon by the malpractice insurance carrier needing to know every legal detail in order to find out a way to escape compensatory damages? Why wasn't the patient and his family sued for not reading the drug package insert? Had any body done so, their eyes would "pop out like stars, and nobody would take the drug! As it turned out via the "grapevine of scuttle but," the patient didn't die, did sustain some kidney damage and was awarded a million dollars.

Dr. David Rubsmasen, who for all I know has horns emerging from each temple, says, according to Assemblyman now Congressman Henry Waxman, nobody can figure out the "compensible event" with a no-fault insurance plan. Politically both agree there's no way to "finance no fault" except with immense difficulty. Under the present arrangement the young man who suffered kidney damage received too much. The dermatologist and the pharmacist should have received something to help them recover from the stress and emotional trauma as a gesture so both of them might live longer! (Don't policemen and sheriffs and firemen, and others, go out on "stress leaves," well compensated? If you don't think being a physician is tougher than being either a policeman or fireman you are really mistaken! You have got to be kidding! It's life and death every day for a physician compared to once in awhile for others facing the problems of society!)

With the system remaining in place prosecuting lawyers can hardly wait to get into these kinds of actions. Some head to "trial lawyers school" in Wyoming to practice shouting and strutting under the auspices of a colorful famous lawyer. Emerging from such dramatic training and bursting with confidence the lawyer looks forward to being able to keep the penthouse suite, maybe even pay off their spouse's credit card(s)! At last focusing on this "evil drug firm" in a courtroom they have that opportunity to swagger in an Italian silk suit in front of a petite jury of 12, all carefully selected by a psychologist who examined each juror's reaction to Italian silk prior to approval.

This jury of 12, not really able to grasp completely what's really going on and who collectively know zero or less about the history of drugs and medical care, may decide upon a reward in the many millions of dollars against the pharmaceutical manufacturer. This jury award, media televised, instills a "vague mistrust in the particular pharmaceutical firm" by the dermatologist and the pharmacist. Why else were they both put through hell on earth? The firm must have done something wrong, should have made a more perfect molecule.

There was a case when even the trial judge failed to escape damnation, wishing he had guided the whole proceedings better. He reeled the evening of the conclusion of the trial. His girl friend criticized the way he handled the proceedings, even denying him sex. He forgot she once worked as an executive for a drug company and won an award for a paper titled, "Paul Ehrlich; Chemotherapy is Launched!"

So, are we going to continue to allow pharmaceutical firms to develop and manufacture medicines? Are we going to continue to let physicians decide who should take medications? Don't you think physicians should take a stand? Why do physicians just roll over for lawyers?

Why have so many new physicians tuned in to "commercialism?" More specifically, why is a medicine that worked wonders in 1960 unable to work the same wonders now?   Why do physicians tell patients who ask about an older drug "No that's an old drug. You should take this 'new' one," especially since he has no experience with the old drug and very little if any with the new?

We are getting close to a "Horn and Hardardt Automat" kind of situation. Instead of a ham and cheese sandwich, the patron sees behind the glass "a little green football shaped tablet, 10mg called Prozac." He thinks as his paper money slips easily through the slot, "I'll try that today because I think I heard it raises "serotonin," and everybody needs more serotonin," or, he sees a "yellow elongated tablet, 300mg named Zantac, not such a big deal. A college student recognizes a very pale "small yellow pill," 10mg.named Aricept. Remembering his mom saying his dad was told he might have "Alzheimer's," and that his dad seemed better on one such Aricept a day, the student imagines it might help him take his finals! Considering if one made dad's thinking better, two ought to help even more, he takes two Aricept tablets then suddenly needs to leave the testing room due to acute diarrhea! He's lucky. Someone else, more brilliant yet and already on three medications, buys a fourth behind the glass to at last cure his toenail fungus. He dies from a drug mixture that caused a cardiac complication called torsade de pointes! Another nearly identical case, rescued that evening by paramedics anxious to please ER doctors loading up expensive hospital intensive care units with as many patients as possible, survives "mindless!" But, with great financial luck his insurance pays the bill of $185000. Well, so much then for selecting your own medications. Both my ears ring to this day hearing this comment some years ago from a guest on educational television's "Wall Street Week." He exclaims, "America is 'still' under medicated."   Horn and Hardardt, here we come!   What kind of insurance will Horn and Hardardt be able to afford, and how much will that influence the price of the drug products?

As for "fixing health care," there was this amusing discussion I had many years ago with a British neurosurgeon of London's famed Queen's Square. What he said really struck me. Moreover the reasons prompting his comment raised my curiosity. On the subject of seemingly mismanaged or over managed patients in America, he replied, "It's your bloody stupid (!) American medical school education!" Medical school education in America has indeed been faltering in terms of clinical expertise. "The tendency to 'not think' about your patient carefully, and 'not time' the procedure you propose with the best interest of the patient in mind," has been a huge consumer problem. Why is everybody's schedule more important than the patient's condition schedule? Ordering far too many "bloody stupid lab tests" and too often relying on "misleading drug levels" has helped cause an unhealthy trend that lacks good sense.

What's really helpful for teaching medical students are those real, live, cooperative hospitalized patients. Simulation of real illness by actors faking disease falls short. There are so many conditions even Marlon Brando couldn't mimick! Teaching medical students etiquette as they relate with "patient actors" perhaps has merit. But are medical students nowadays abrasive with people by nature? Think about it! Isn't it better to ask a live teaching case to please allow a medical student to look him over even if it means being worked up several times?

There are too many medical students being trained nowadays, in my opinion. There are way too many homeless citizens! As mentioned in chapter one voter registration records reveal many homeless may be located where the form indicated on certain cross streets where NW, NE, SW, SE indicates their regular location at that corner of the block. How is it so many simply fall through the cracks only to live this way? Would free medical care from trainees spoil their day? Would medical students get more experience seeing homeless rather than actors?

Making arrangements for homeless who cooperate, getting them all cleaned up imagine how many different kinds of illnesses are going to be seen. Scabies is one (how does an actor fake scabies?). A rare Wegener's mid line granuloma may rarely show itself (how's an actor going to fake that?). Signs of under nutrition and alcoholism are virtually guaranteed. There are "spent shells from drug abuse" and conceivably a variety of presenting illnesses that could never be experienced through medical student-actor inter relationships and video evaluations. Well paid members of teaching staffs too often prefer evaluating private patients for additional income, or their research project to keep funds coming in, or going to court to testify for an extra pay check much more than teaching medical students. At least these seem the reasons why actors in recent years have become part of medical student teaching programs. If it's not the case from what I've heard, I apologize!

Newer and different doesn't necessarily mean better. The nineteen fifties medical school education remains hard to beat because it deals with essential basics. Molecular biology and immunology may be studied after medical school from a book. So much happening, there is no escape anyway from a lifetime of study for any physician looking forward to practicing good medicine today. It's essential to keep up on what's happening should your patients ask about what they've heard, even though nothing discussed can be applied for years to come. Having knowledge increases confidence.

In the mid nineteen sixties there was interest in phasing out the general practitioner emphasizing all physicians pick an area of interest, study it and specialize. Emerging was "immunology," which addressed illnesses ranging from the common cold to multiple sclerosis to all forms of cancer. Immunology was immunology whatever you needed to better understand and treat. Even if too soon to provide a needed treatment per se, it provided practitioners willing to study knowledge leading to an vastly improved way to explain illness to patients.

In research, the fruit fly (drosophila melanogaster) was familiar to all pre medical students. It quickly became the favorite for genetic experiments, especially mutations that proceeded a million times faster than in humans. The fruit fly, however, had no immune system. It was discovered the mouse had an immune system much like a human, at least in a very basic respect, thus mice gradually became favorite experimental animals. And thus far no groups have gathered for street demonstrations against experiments with mice.

For a short time the feeling was all forms of cancer were due to viruses. That was dispelled by physician researchers J. Michael Bishop MD and Harold E. Varmus MD at UCSF who became Nobel Prize laureates in medicine in 1989. A mutated gene, their "oncogene" for example one on chromosome 17 called "p53" was shown involved in over half of all human cancers! Oncogenes can work in concert mysteriously causing cancer. A retrovirus, actually a family of RNA viruses with enzymatic ability to transform and incorporate within the DNA of cells, can incite oncogene(s) to cause cancer. As a result using "retrovirus transport for gene therapy" must give pause regarding safety.

The time had come for the specialist to start studying regularly to keep up with concepts. How was a busy general practitioner going to find time to do that, and if not, then what? The alternative was to become "dumb," "dumber," or dumbest!" as knowledge burgeons.

The public however expressed this great desire for a "family" doctor. The American Academy of "Family" Practice responded. Were they going to give up the easy money? Typically it was the "family doctor" that referred patients to surgeons. It was the family doctor that usually got to be surgical assistant to pick up a handsome fee for doing next to nothing, or, in fact, not even being necessary to the trained surgeon. This "conflict of interest" was typically ignored. Such practice continued for decades. "Family" doctors played the role of "ghost surgeons," the actual surgeon performing the surgery not even personally known to the patient. The real surgeon received the most pay though not the most credit. Of course there were general practitioners that had natural talent for surgery, however, in measured terms of specialty training they were not "qualified." ("Being certified got political by the end of the nineteen sixties whereby being qualified was determined by where and how long you were trained.)

My favorite example of an exception was Charles F. Nelson, the first physician in Beverly Hills. A surgical specialist that assisted Dr. Nelson at California hospital in Los Angeles told me he often had trouble keeping up with him admitting he just had the skills. Charles' initials, "CF" were also known as "calcium fixation" and he involved himself with lab experiments in mice focusing on calcium. Of course his therapeutic "long and short calcium IV treatments may have been mostly placeboes," but, make no mistake Dr. Nelson and his thoughts about therapeutics were ahead of his time. I knew him quite well and can say if all general practitioners were like Charles, there would be fewer specialists. I spent two weeks with CF Nelson as a senior medical student. For my "missionary externship as a senior medical student, I wisely chose "Beverly Hills!"

Another problem that defied improvement was the strict compartmentalization of specialties. Everyone had his "turf" and God help the practitioner who invaded another specialist's turf! The famed albeit tragic Nork case in Sacramento was the first big example. Neurosurgeons were already doing far too much unnecessary back surgery, which they finally admitted. When Dr. Nork, an orthopedist (!), began doing the same thing and with a neurosurgeon assistant to boot named Hal Holland! this raised the roof. Dr. Holland also made a study of confounding the defense in various courtrooms more than one malpractice case with examples typical for the prosecutable side.   That alone was enough to aggravate many doctors. I was asked by "the attorney" picked to bring Nork down to help him with anatomy of the spinal column using a cadaver. I Refused. It was a surprise medico-legal-politics had progressed to such a point.. I knew Nork by virtue of seeing some cases for him. I knew Holland, seeing cases for him. I eventually saw "Nork victims" following the 50million collective malpractice jury awards disaster that bankrupted Liberty Mutual Medical Malpractice Insurance for 23 northern California counties! This colossal mess stemmed from what followed as those opposing Nork had a trial moved to San Francisco. "OW Jones, MD," the famed San Francisco neurosurgeon, was persuaded to testify against Nork. That did it! An avalanche of negligence compensations followed one after the other. It was said Nork "mishandled tissues surgically" but it's very doubtful that rumor was true.

The Miofski malpractice case of Sacramento that also drained the malpractice insurance pool was pathetic and bizarre. I knew Miofski a little, practicing in Sacramento, at least to the extent of having a pleasant lunch with him at Sutter General Hospital. An anesthesiologist, my guess he was sniffing inhalants used for hospital surgical cases. He was misusing and taking drugs with three other physicians of Sacramento from the same medical school back east. A psychiatrist should have been alerted from the start to avert a ludicrous situation that went on six months before "a nurse blew the whistle that cost her job," and reportedly resulted in the chief of staff of Sutter Memorial hanging himself!" For months physicians around town were laughing over rumors about Miofski and his cases. Miofski unsuccessfully attempted suicide in a motel and subsequently was placed in a mental facility. All was preventable and not funny at all. Miofski's debauchery was de facto harmless because the patients were unaware and under anesthesia. The publicity, however, ruined people. For the record I was in Laguna Beach California when this went on. Thirty or so patients from Sacramento continued follow up visits with me in Laguna Beach. There was talk and bad publicity about The Miofski case and information I received was a reiteration of this tragic set of circumstances.

Opposing so much specialty compartmentalization by 1970 a concerted interest was created devoted to "muscle." It began in Philadelphia with the "muscle biology club." General physicians paid little attention but specialists didn't either. "Muscle" however, meant skeletal muscle, the heart muscle, extra ocular muscles and the smooth non-striated muscles that made up "all the sacs (stomach, uterus) and tubes (bowel) within the human body!" A heart, eye or GI specialist was not, however, about to request consultation from an "expert on muscle." The very idea of a specialty on muscle overlapping specialties was politically unacceptable, however, one should not underestimate the value.

A gynecologist from Illinois was the one who measured uterine sac pressures during pre menstrual cramping. He previously recorded a pressure of 15mm of mercury within a relaxed uterus. Measurements as high as 180mm of mercury were recorded before a menstrual period explaining "why" the terrific cramping pain! This led to a breakthrough with the non-steroid anti-inflammatory drug, ibuprofen (Motrin) that opposes certain prostaglandins (lipids) to foster uterine smooth muscle relaxation at the critical time. Regardless psychologists and PMS specialists continued to make a nice living since many insist on making the syndrome much more complicated, and of course it was! A diuretic was often indicated for fluid retention and "bad behavior!" PMS specialists still thrived.

Buy the nineteen seventies the "family" physician was extolled as the only physician that was truly "holistic!" This seemed strange. Even a "pipe line heart surgeon," who did nothing more than replace mitral or aortic heart valves every Tuesday, was holistic. Had you talked with the heart surgeon you discover he's aware if he did a perfect job the patient, spouse, family and the relatives all would benefit. Wasn't that being holistic?

"Wholeness" meaning above and beyond the fundamental parts (e.g. the heart valves) composing touchable reality stemmed from Gestalt psychology of the nineteen thirties. In America it was a means opposing scientific analytical approaches that overlooked human values in general. The psychiatrists and psychologists were "specialists!" How did the general practitioners get involved? It was the publics' vote that did it!

Interpreting phenomena as organized wholes begins with Max Wertheimer, Kurt Koffka and Wolfgang Kohler in the nineteen twenties. DNA Nobel Laureate biophysicist Francis Crick of the Salk Institute continues the challenge but stays the course to understand the brain through in depth examination of how the brain "sees" pushing still further determining how and why we are "conscious?" Charles Gilbert, Rockefellar U., New York, and VS Ramachandran, famous psychologist of UC San Diego who also explores brain function along with my long time friend Oliver Sacks MD, head neurologist at Belleview Hospital in New York City, labor to interpret phenomena as organized wholes. Having known or at least brushed elbows with such "geniuses," I depend upon them to help the neurologist such as myself understand the brain. As "a supposed expert" (officially) and having done psychiatry 25 years for California, as a neurologist for 40years with an interest in the brain 49 years I'm still very short explaining the brain or "especially the mind." As Crick has so aptly pointed out there much more to learn! The truth I'm delighted to know a little bit about it.

Brain disease once termed "functional" has been pinned down in terms of specific electrical-chemical disturbances at the molecular level. Better ways of explaining delusions and hallucinations have been arrived at and thus improved ideas for treatment. Up to 1990 virtually nothing was known concerning the biological, neurological or chemical basis of consciousness or memory. On 1/27/03 it was a pleasure to listen to Francis Crick's long time friend, Jack Cowan, professor of mathematics at the University of Chicago lecture on his "mathematical struggle," to utilize power laws and exponent differences to liken brain neuron firing patterns to that of a forest fire.

Tragically, during the nineteen nineties with the popularity of surgical transplantation procedures, a body part became worth more than a human life. For money a college student was left to die after being kidnapped and relieved of a kidney. As medical care became a business it got to be like a concept of "auto salvage," whereby all parts sold separately amounted to much more than the cost of a new vehicle. Physicians as well as patients had better not conceptualize medical care along lines of "arbitrage and junk bonds." (That would be the antithesis of Gestalt holism.)

Physicians are not going to be perfect and neither are patients. But it's immensely important that both hang on to their ideals. For physicians to do this a despicable situation where physicians ready for practice have overwhelming debt must be addressed. A physician deeply in debt is without a choice not to become part of a discombobulated third party health care insurance system that also includes the hospital.

A big leap forward to improve care consists of doing away with malpractice politics and putting in place ARBITRATION. True, one gives up the right to bring forth an action for money but much is gained in return for society. For starters there is no reason to tamper with patients medical files under such a system of no-fault. Secondly caution is given more consideration on the part of the physician and the patient. A more thoughtful kind of doctor-patient relationship begins. By replacing our tort system, so lethargic and injurious, with arbitration then reasonable compensation for damage, loss of license, and fraud can be reduced. More idealistic physicians are going to be less likely to give up and quit. A hospital with too many bad "apples," if it is closed down, will at least be closed for the right reason.

There's always room for a good doctor or a good lawyer? Isn't it a fact there are too many in both professions? What's wrong with vacating one graduating class in a teaching institution? What's wrong with reducing the size of classes? Has rational sociological thinking been blocked by obsessions for funds, grants, bloated living wills, or money and nothing but money when adjustments could be made to do with less?

Fifty states may have 50 different ideas. The situation collectively worsens. For medical care to improve for everyone there needs to be a central authority. It's like banking. In fact medical centers and hospitals are managed financially by banks! A reliable "predictable way" for physicians getting paid promptly for services is essential. Medical care must also be made available for all citizens. You mustn't leave sick people to die and say you're part of a civilized society. When former president Bill Clinton held that proposed medical care card up before congress, entitling everyone to medical care, as part of his first State of the Union Message you had to know if you're really a doctor, that's the way it should be.

Before Rome fell, Rome was very successful through exertion of central authority. All roads led to Rome. As the great empire divided into four parts, two East and two West, it became too stretched out. Local failures became inevitable. With loss of central authority gradually the worst kind of politics prevailed, namely "local politics." The United States has revealed evidence of its' shortcomings; properly organized medical care for its' masses among them. America where medical care is concerned remains steadily more divided, not just into four parts, two East and two West, like "Rome," but "50." For some time now it has seemed time to unite and pull together.

CHAPTER III

HOSPITALS AS EMPLOYERS – SO MANY PROBLEMS!

Three of Plato's seven virtues are "Christian," namely faith, hope and charity. The virtues of Judaism are the same and, having traveled the world a little and meeting those of Islamic faith, Buddhists and others, it seems rather obvious to me the major religions of the world all endorse "faith," "hope," and "charity." Those that embrace some other form of religion have somehow endorsed a rewrite of their own scriptures.

Hospitals in America are named after Catholic Saints and then there is Barnes Jewish Hospital in St. Louis Missouri. There's a Hoag Presbyterian Hospital in Newport Beach California and the Methodist Hospital in Oklahoma City. Being admitted to a hospital anywhere in our United States, it's just as important today as before the "age of penicillin" to maintain hope and faith. However, most everyone knows not to expect "charity," because there is very little if any, not any more.

Whether you prefer to think like a biological engineer (molecular biologist), or as a psychoanalyst MD, experiences in life sooner or later convince you what Karl Meninger said, "The toughest thing in life can be adjusting to a 'loss'." Within any area where a hospital is still considered essential the population of the region is forced to adjust to this inhospitable loss of charity. Ivory tower medical teaching centers, as well as major hospitals within the United States, are managed financially by banks. To survive, bankers must focus virtually all of their attention on one thing, "making money!" However, it is very interesting to discover how a large bank, such as the Bank of America, operating like all member banks on discounted loans and customers' deposits, decides to simply write off millions of dollars. In certain situations you might be shocked to learn ten million dollars is not worth bothering about. The Board votes, "Let's just write it off. All in favor say yes. Good! It's unanimous."

Where the human condition is concerned relating especially to hospital based medical care in the United States, it is presently split into two extremes. Both extremes have to do with banking. On the one hand what's perceived rightly or wrongly as an emergent medical matter may be taken in immediately under Medicare and supplemental insurance, especially if you are over 65 years of age with such a prospect of the hospital raking in big money! On the other hand in the HMO more structured hospital situation, citing Kaiser-Permanente as the best of "structured care" (medicine managed by lawyers and accountants), if the perceived emergent matter is "truly emergent," you may find it difficult to be taken care of very quickly. It's "let's go for it and make money" in the first instance versus a "stall to perhaps save some expenditures" in the latter instance, both dealing with what's perceived by laity as something that needs attention right away.

If you have never been acutely ill before and belong to an HMO and "don't know the ropes," you could die or be robbed of all quality of life before you are properly evaluated and treated. This happens, sadly enough, even though the Kaiser HMO for certain has both physician expertise and the procedural ability to handle your case! For one thing you typically are going to be reluctant to impose yourself upon the system, or you simply don't know to present yourself at their ER doorstep. Why? You are not aware you are that sick! As an acute patient you are unaware of how much time you have left. Example: how would you know if suddenly an Epstein Barr virus activates causing you to think you have the "flu," when in fact you have a warm antibody hemolytic anemia that can kill you just as fast as black water fever from falciparum malaria? Even the most astute specialist having a good day may be thrown off on that one! What doctor is always prepared for "that presentation?" How many lawyers are going to be anxious to sue should the doctor miss that diagnosis? Luckily such presentations are not common, otherwise HMOs would change their ways. Uncommon things are uncommon.

With the one example you are sucked right in, saved, then bankrupted! In the other instance you are stonewalled by the "rules of the appointment process." Under managed care you may be stonewalled at any age. Under private care, if you are under age 65 and unable to afford insurance like 45 million Americans, diagnosis and treatment costs not uncommonly necessitate a second home mortgage should you own a home and plan to pay the outrageous bill. There's the threat of bankruptcy for anyone in business. No consideration is given to a fact employees will automatically lose their jobs should their business be bankrupted by medical costs for the boss or any member of his or her family. (Of course you can always threaten the CEO of a hospital, or the chancellor of a medical center, to lower charges if you know exactly how to do it without being hauled off by the county sheriff.)

What saves the HMO is that most presenting conditions thought to be very urgent are not urgent. There is usually enough time, most things are taken care of and most everyone eventually is happy with their plan. The stresses of modern life create a host of physiological symptoms that may mimic a great variety of pathological conditions. Statistically, however, a few people are going to die that didn't have to die. What preserves the hospital system governed by Medicare is an ability to deal with acute conditions quickly. The Medicare-private system is more apt to save the very unusual surprise case while collecting huge amounts of money from those sources to compensate for those who can't pay, don't pay, run off and won't pay, or qualify as a write off.

A case of polymyalgia rheumatica hospitalized in 1963 costs $250. The same case today with the same treatment, prednisone, costs $30,000! Such a peculiar case whereby a 65 years old cannot flex their hips or raise their arms because of excruciating pain responds dramatically to an initial dose of 100mg prednisone, best tapered systematically to zero within ten days. Without complications in two months the patient who entered the ward by stretcher may be back to normal! There is no need to even hospitalize the patient if you're positive of the diagnosis. Try to convince a patient or family of that! In the hospital over staffed many physicians get to see this strange condition. And rarely if complications occur, such as inflammation of arterial channels, then it gets much more expensive. Such a case becomes valuable for "hospital business." Such cases support the "system." Insurance payments allow a hospital to pay its employees and obligations. Employment countrywide is of the utmost importance to the welfare of the nation.

Many physicians are called in to evaluate hospital cases based upon patient responses to admitting nurse's notes. "Do you have blurry vision?" If you reply, "Maybe occasionally," that will be sufficient to have your eyes checked by an ophthalmologist! The ophthalmologist may call in a retinologist over some question or suspicion for the beginning of a detached retina! Suspicion of a hemorrhoid may call for a proctologist. Heartburn may call for a cardiologist or a specialist for stomach, intestinal and other abdominal organ disorders. Physicians are sold on the idea of sharing cases with other physicians that have the same malpractice carrier. There's such a fear of malpractice any physician outside the loop may be suspected as someone who might testify against you should you carry out a plan and make a mistake. Policy for specialists is determined by committee decisions. Focus is also on what's best "financially" for the hospital, and how best to "defend" the hospital.

The days of relying on stethoscopes and taking time to obtain a "good medical history and physical examination" are past. There's a lot more money to be made with sophisticated high-tech instrumentation. General Electric and SonoSite Corporations offer machines that cost in the tens of thousands of dollars to replace a $100 stethoscope! Medical students are no longer encouraged to spend enough time to practice with a stethoscope. "The length and quality of the tubing is extremely important!" Stethoscopes sold for $40 are usually worthless and many such are sold for home use. They're used by those who have little idea what they are doing, what they're hearing or what they're measuring. A few cardiologists, as part of educational programs, are paid to lecture disparagingly about using stethoscopes touting new technology that picks up everything as if to say physicians using stethoscopes might as well be "deaf and dumb." Why bother with a stethoscope when you can use a portable hand held ultrasound machine for $55000? Instead of having a listen you may conveniently carry this equipment in a small case and have a comprehensive look at a patient's major internal organs. What this can lead to is anybody's guess since the interpretation of ultrasound findings is going to also be a guess until you become an expert. Being unsure of what you are visualizing the patient then is likely to be "hospitalized!" One thing for certain all such attempts to become involved with high tech procedures creates a potential for much more expense, something nobody needs. Medical care and medication costs have already encroached upon many a patient's budget allotted for housing and food!

Mammography remains extremely popular even though eighty percent of breast tumors are discovered by palpation! Palatial mammography centers, much more so than centers offering thermograms (regional temperature difference maps), are highly advertised and desired by most all women. It doesn't matter ten million cancer cells fit on the head of a straight pin! Do you think someone is going to detect 100,000 cells? Repeat testing due to uncertainties just adds to the anxiety. Women have their breasts removed due to inaccurate interpretations. Unnecessary tests still generate payments to private investors or to those large insurance companies that "sell high-tech equipment on credit" or better yet lease it to hospitals. Hospital insurance carrier costs are sky high, and remain about sixty percent of sky high with the requirement you must insure the hospital bed that's empty! Management's desire is logically directed towards filling that bed! The number of employees of hospitals automatically increases with need for technical assistance to manage various kinds of scanners and other equipment. Employees must be paid enough to live close enough to the hospital to get to work on time. They can't afford a helicopter! Higher management requires the same and they command very high salaries. It is true their positions are demanding.

There is a huge expense for "malpractice defense" not simply for physicians but for the nurses and the hospital as well. The legal profession, with hardly a dearth of lawyers, continually aims for any situation that can be shaped into wrongdoing, using "deep pocket," and "wrongful death" arguments to their very best advantage. When lawyers can't convince a physician to testify against another physician even for a substantial amount of money they find a Ph.D. happy to testify against a physician to help make their case.

There's no benefit to society to allow a hospital or a reputable firm to go bankrupt because of some unbelievably extravagant jury award. If you have 100 serious problems in a hospital doing quite well, and one case of elective cosmetic surgery that unexpectedly goes sour resulting in a negligence action, lobbying efforts may be made to put such legal action in perspective. Because of the magnitude of the threat judges are made aware of such circumstances. Some effort to maintain rational balance must be made. How could it be otherwise?

Jurors are easily influenced by the sway of proceedings in a courtroom. During the course of a physician-on-trial for negligence, any juror excused for illness to see their doctor may be influenced by a comment from that doctor, especially if the doctor on trial is a target of a medical society. This constitutes "jury tampering of the most subtle kind." Any physician in legal trouble the hospital typically dissociates itself from that physician even though up to that point he or she was a reputable member of the staff. The hospital must maintain its community image! Across the nation physicians prostitute themselves for money. "Everyone has a right to make a living," comes now the reason. They sell predictable plaintiff or defense testimony to throw one side or the other off balance. As long ago as the nineteen sixties it was $500 to testify, $1500 to lie. Imagine the amounts paid now! To settle compensation cases, hospitalized or not, physician's licenses are virtually purchased! In other words a form is filled out and the physician simply signs at the bottom of the form. By eliminating psychiatric factors that are bound to play a substantial role, especially job injury cases lasting over a year (!), such cases may then be quickly settled. It's just statistics.

Employees of a hospital like any workers who employ devious means to be relieved from work need a physician's approval. A tentative diagnosis must "fit a computer program for payment" and may not reflect the truth. Underlying may be need for relief because of mental cruelty from higher management or, a psychiatric matter and/or a sociological-economic reason in which case the settlement becomes a type of welfare payment. Sometimes divorce complicates the situation with consideration then for the welfare of parents and their children. Sometimes there's a mentally ill child that compromises the employee's ability to function normally at work. The employee, exhausted, is ashamed to mention this type of situation. In short it is a complicated (!) world we live in. What appears fraudulent may not be purposeful malingering. When you carefully examine the entire situation and what goes on behind the scenes a reasonable temporary solution may be achieved that makes sense when all factors are considered. Of course there is that "injury at play" that is claimed as an "injury at work." What would you do? It's all part of socialism within the framework of capitalism.

The medical profession over decades has gradually involved itself in a snarl with the legal profession and the insurance industry. "All out combat for money" has been on the increase. Wrongdoing has been apparent everywhere you look. Price gauging, duplicate pricing, overcharging, unpredictable charging, fraudulent practices, cover up, mistrust, over utilization, all represent just part of the list of misbehavior. A close examination of what's wrong in such a tangle of inter personal relationships reflects "narcissism."

Corporate America now includes hospitals and medical centers and therein is excessive entitlement and exploitation. There's the taking advantage of others to achieve one's ends. There's a pervasive preoccupation with unlimited success, power together with a lack of empathy, or unwillingness, to identify with the feelings of others. Instead there is the focus of attention on an image of self and the institution to which "you have given your life!" What's more extraordinary it all seems acceptable today as simply "the American way!" It narrows down to cases of a narcissistic personality envying another, neither one seemingly aware of it. America is too very haughty nowadays and this is recognized overseas. It is not in the best interest of "the land of the free and home of the brave." Americans should be liked and respected instead of envied because of a conviction we all have so much money. Too many are on the rock pile trying to afford their wants.

As for hospitals one philosophical way to look at all this is to not be concerned in the least. If neither hospitals nor physicians existed the human species would survive! Those seriously ill that could have been saved would die. Certain persons would live even longer since the risk of hospitalization is eliminated. There are no hospitals! Those lucky enough to escape serious illness and injury, and who escape harm of all kinds, would not be affected at all and need not care. Someone is still going to live to be 100.

On the other hand physicians and hospitals are meant to be part of civilization. Logician historian of Oxford Arnold Toynbee argues no civilization survives without interpersonal relationships (the sum of which defines that society within a given population) continuing to demonstrate good will. Civilizations fall as the sum of destructive behavior (lack of civility) increases sufficiently to abolish this quintessential ingredient. Granted, there are those who are persuaded that "Rome fell because of lead poisoning." This however is tantamount to saying America is now failing as a young civilization because of "fumes." There may be some lead, and there may be some fumes, but these aren't the reasons!

In spite of all are troubles and conflicts absolutely amazing medical and surgical procedures heretofore unimagined are now available. This is what is so emphasized by the political arm of organized medicine, and rightly so! These achievements, however, are not available to patients due to the brilliance of medical politicians anxious to control all the nation's doctors, but rather by a few outstanding determined individuals that showed they could do something exceptional, went ahead and pulled it off!

Check this (!): some people are born with abnormal heart conduction pathways. As a teenager their heartbeat may jump off track and suddenly slow to 20 beats a minute or suddenly beat 200 beats per minute for no apparent reason whatsoever! This impossible situation, once one of the worst nightmares to face any practicing cardiologist, may be "curable" (yes, cured!) within just the past ten years. With development of the IV drug Adenogard, then using medications time proven for open-heart surgery to relax the heart (Versed, Fentenyl and Phenergan), the most tedious procedure imaginable is undertaken. It involves special catheters exploring through veins (not arteries, but thin walled veins!). There takes place a methodical search for the exact location of the abnormal cardiac conduction pathway repeatedly signaling the "hunter' by stimulation of the abnormal heartbeats those abnormal beats temporarily eliminated with Adenogard with a 10 second half-life. After hours of searching for the culprit pathway it is, at last, zeroed in! It is then put out of commission, forever, via microwave technology! For the pioneer cardiologist who did all this when the tops in the field figured he'd never make it (not every cardiologist can do this, remember that!), a parade consisting of many of his grateful patients took place in his city in the late nineteen nineties. Take a bow doctor, "break a leg!"

Heart surgeons today actually repair a grossly disfigured (mitral) heart valve. Unable to snap shut tightly, if the valve is not repaired, it needs to be replaced. A very successful high profile movie celebrity had a normal pulmonary valve removed and put in place of his worn out aortic valve. His pulmonary artery valve was then replaced with a very successful makeshift valve product. This amazing procedure was done via a small opening in his chest at USC medical center in Los Angeles! Three years later in 2003 the celebrity is doing fine. It's really amazing, but so is the cost of the hospitalization!

Hip and knee replacements are now performed to perfection by many skilled orthopedists, fulfilling what was no more than an "orthopedist's pipe dream in the nineteen fifties." There used to be so much painful suffering tolerated for too long by patients with necrosis of the neck of the femur, and with bum knees. Football players are very grateful. Some hospitals use ultra violet light to help curb infections with reported good success. What cost $25000 ten years ago may now cost $50000! Where are the limits of affordability for these procedures requiring a hospital setting?

For the masses the overwhelming problem is one of affordability for the essential hospitalization and procedure(s). Ablation of the abnormal heart conduction pathway priced at about $15000 during the nineties still remains within reach of nearly everyone whether a car salesman or a super rich Arab oil sheik. But many wonderful procedures are so expensive they can put a middle class working family in debt for life, or at least with costs high enough to rob their children of a chance to be helped financially to get a college education. And you must pay the hospital bill like paying a bank.

Occasionally, hospitals and hospital based surgeons do perform a "write off," should the patient be one of what organized medicine refers to as "one of the working poor." This pejorative description is about people who work regularly, are able to purchase food, clothing and transportation, and to successfully make a monthly condo payment. But, they own no property that can be profitably attached! Should that type person drop to the sidewalk and receive ambulance transportation to a hospital and receive coronary artery by pass surgery, if determined necessary, the bill could reach $100,000. Who knows for certain?

If you own property the bank representing the hospitals' obligations will dispose of your property to pay their bills. Hospitals may be among the top three employers in towns, cities or counties. The payroll must be met! Elderly rest home patients even unaware of their surroundings and waiting to die peacefully are admitted with acute conditions under Medicare to support hospital financial needs. The same scenario occurs with retarded illness. Someone with an IQ of 40 and physical disabilities seemingly denying any quality of life are admitted to intensive care for treatment of a superimposed acute condition. Lawyers enforce this policy. Nurses break down and cry servicing such patients. It's worse than any scene from a horror movie. The reason of course is to cover the bottom line.

Most physicians are motivated to be part of this great profession for reasons besides money. No matter how skilled or dedicated all become locked firmly within a "system." None can do anything about it. It's essentially controlled by hospital policy. Most citizenry never become sick enough to get a view of some of the uncivilized goings on. President Bill Clinton is the first since Harry Truman to use the bully pulpit to cry out that America's medical care system "needs fixing," offering specific suggestions to at least make things better for everyone. Truman and Clinton, both very good presidents of the US, got all beat up! Truman ducks bullets on the steps of Blair House. Former president Reagan is geared to push for such reforms. As chance would have it he instead gets shot and nearly killed by a schizophrenic! President Gerald Ford is I believe another inclined to push for medical care improvements but he too was shot at having to duck bullets in Sacramento and San Francisco California! I vouch for Reagan because of personal conversation with him. I vouch for Ford having never met him because why else would Bob Hope like him so much, and then there's the Betty Ford Clinic!

Why don't congressmen and senators do something? It's a matter of maintaining employment. Our system of capitalism demands this. Our nation with obvious tendencies towards monopoly, not just fair competition, is in part responsible for creating our discombobulated socialism. The United States needs growth and it needs its working force to pay taxes. Sadly people of America continue to forget what president Nixon said about "tearing up those 'credit' cards." Personal debt is now so high people wince at the idea of paying more taxes. The rather miraculous achievement of a balanced budget in the late nineteen nineties giving a chance to reduce our debts to other countries is now of the past. This is serious! Ross Perot uses pie charts to point out the interest alone the US owes on the capital sum invested in America by other nations, "betting on our continued prosperity," which is staggering! We can't readily reduce the interest payments without paying down the principle. We are leveraged out! Congressman Chris Cox (R), Newport Beach California issues an annual financial report of where we stand for anyone to read. It's available upon request so why not get hold of a copy and read it? Then it's a matter of "attitude."

Hospital and out-patient "Scanomania" and testing to be "sure" consumes nearly 15% of what the total working force of the US earns annually. Medicines good in the fifties are still good, but oh no, your physician is brainwashed to tell you to be sure and take the "new medication that may be 30 fold more expensive!" Medicare controlled hospitals go right along with the expensive trades. HMO Kaiser-Permanente sensibly figures if a medication is useful in the sixties why isn't it useful now? If our genes are the same as thirty years ago why is it only some new medicine is going to work? What is wrong with cheaper medicines that worked wonders back then? That's easy to answer! There's less profit!

In or out of the hospital it's best to start with a very low dosage of a prescribed medication (of course there are in hospital indications to do otherwise though not as a rule with outpatients), observing and asking how the patient feels as the dosage is raised. Instead physicians often prescribe a "macho dose" to start that causes the patient to reel with side effects easily avoided. Hearing the alarming news the physician switches and prescribes another expensive drug and repeats the same mistake! Physicians order drug levels suspecting a patient (or the nurse) is at fault. More money is spent! Billions of dollars are spent needlessly that would not be spent if beginning prescriptions were conservative. Patients get into car wrecks taking more medicine than they need. This is nuts, isn't it? Doesn't anybody get it? Too much medicine gets people hospitalized! It becomes a merry go round of prescription stupidity.

Unnecessary things are done in hospitals to support too many doctors of all kinds leasing offices near the hospital in buildings either owned by the hospital or long time doctors on the hospital staff. All physicians, as part of the hospital staff, need to make those lease payments! Numerous consultations, X-ray studies, heart testing, lung testing, all sorts of testing and pathology laboratory equipment are continually over utilized all supervised by "physician concessionaires." It's like selling hot dogs at the Rose Bowl and it is what's known as "peanut stand medicine," a term used with a chuckle by this New York internist I knew in the late sixties.

Sadly the inability of American researchers to find the cause of AIDs, depending upon the French group at the Pasteur in Paris to do it, resulted in an AIDs epidemic among the homosexual and unclean needle street drug population that hit like a ton of bricks. Somehow money needed to improve blood bank screening failed to materialize within a most helpful time frame. The prevalence of opportunistic disease due to critically diminished numbers of signal calling lymphocytes (T-cells) incapacitated by the tiny retro-virus, typical of such presentations, led to expensive pharmacological treatment and procedures including very expensive brain surgery. The financial drain that affected others needing hospitalization along with their insurance carriers, due to medical, social and political demands to address an AIDs disaster, proved nevertheless a boost to hospital coffers.

On rare occasion diagnostic stupidity, personified, led to an extremely favorable outcome for a hospitalized patient as medical staff bungled its way along unwittingly, ultimately doing the patient some real benefit! A lady was admitted to hospital with chest discomfort, her general physician not observing her hyperventilating from anxiety. His concern focused on heartburn. Nurse's notes revealed she had occasional inner left knee pain and considerable trouble walking because of the pain. An orthopedist was called in who found absolutely nothing wrong with the patient's knees. Privately he thought she was a "nut." A routine PAP smear was obtained with a suspiciously positive comment on the report. A gynecologist was summoned for what he figured was just a quick routine pelvic check and a handsome fee for just a couple minutes work. Low and behold he palpated a pelvic mass consistent with an ovarian cyst! Upon pelvic surgery he discovered a large "chocolate cyst of the ovary!" In his excitement, the cyst burst and fluid sprayed everywhere. Luckily it was a benign adenoma, not malignant, so at least "cancer cells hadn't flown all over the room!" The large cyst was the basis for the patient's knee pain due to pressure on her left obturator nerve. Post op she was able to walk comfortably. The inner left knee pain was gone! A correction in her history revealed it was the worrisome knee pain that contributed to her anxious worrying in the first place. The "heartburn" went away by itself. Sadly her GP failed to pick up on all this till much later since the patient was one of 12 he hospitalized to whom he would say "hello" each morning for a total of $600 daily billings. The patient upon discharge, ever so grateful, has continued to see her GP recommending him as a "wonderful family doctor."

Physicians deserving a lot of blame for contributing to US health cares' downfall early on are those who for some twisted reasoning decided to become attorneys. Most were anesthesiologists who were tired of getting all the blame every time something undesirable happened as a result of surgery. Becoming also a lawyer however was not the best answer for society. In the nineteen sixties hearsay had it neurosurgeons at UCLA with outstanding reputations in Los Angeles were getting sued about once a week! One anesthesiologist-attorney I spoke with in the late sixties had 300 negligence cases going at a given time and Frank Lanterman of the California legislature had evidence about one of his cases sufficient to nail this "doctor-lawyer" who admitted on the phone that he was finally a bit worried.

For sake of hospitals, their staffs and perhaps all of us, to say the legal system in America needs reforming is an understatement. The core of our litigious society consists of a very small percent of the population who suffer delusional thinking short of being schizophrenic. The common law system in the US, now codified, but not like the Code Napoleon, "is an incredibly slow process!" In law there is substance and form. More from lack of fundamental knowledge than intent many legal actions are filed with lack of substance (merit). The lawyer may feel confident he can "teach the jury" at trial. Jurors may be emotionally swayed as in a scapegoat case. Awards can be extremely unrealistic! There is nothing praiseworthy that arises from medical malpractice lawsuits. Such actions never make a better doctor. It is stressful for judges hearing such cases. They wince. Sadly the whole process constitutes hell on earth and all for money.

There are insurance policies for nearly everything because Americans desire insurance protection, so I don't see how "this hatred for insurance companies" is justified. Sociologically it is very wrong to target an insurance company as simply a source of money but there are lawyers doing this regularly for clients who do have the right to bring forth an action. Insurance pool money comes from premium payments and company investment strategies! The principle of insurance is sound. Everyone pays in a small amount so those, hopefully a small number, who suffer a loss can be compensated. I imagine it took thousands of years of interpersonal relationships for societies to come together to realize the good sense of having insurance! Hospitals need insurance. They need insurance for protection from lawsuits, especially malicious mischief, and disproportionate actions that threaten to senselessly close the facility. The hospital, however, also needs your medical coverage insurance money if and when they have that opportunity to get it." The hospital must meet its payroll and obligations that include payments to insurance companies and private investors who have become sponsors of certain equipment (gamma knife or PET scanners for instance) with a profit motive in mind.

Facing these economic circumstances if you are an employee of a large firm that agrees to purchase for employees, 1.5million dollar hospitalization and medical care insurance policies you logically become a "financial target" if and when you become ill and are hospitalized! With a plan providing such a potential large source of money for the hospital you are going to get the best care, and then some! You the patient are in the middle between the hospital needing funds on the one hand and the source of insurance money on the other. Getting as much of that 1.5 million dollars becomes a rationale to do many tests, consultations and procedures. A legitimate hospital charge of $20,000 may become $60,000 even if you are a relatively simple fixable case. There is also a very seamy side to all this that involves "the obviously not fixable case and their families," which I personally brought to the attention of Senator Arlen Specter of Pennsylvania during 1999. Such an example however proved to be no surprise, hard to prove and very sad indeed.

Senator Specter has been very involved for years to improve health care provided some plan that he approves has a chance of passing approval by the senate. I can speak for the senator. If he thought there was reasonable proof some Chinese herb would cure cancers he would soapbox for that herb, at the same time twist the arm of those of the FDA to get it approved! Brought to his office was a detailed example, just one of so many examples, of the not-fixable case. "Such patients have been tortured with tests and procedures every physician who keeps up knows won't help and, in fact, may make the imminent demise of such a patient worse, all in the name of getting as much of 1.5 million dollars as possible. Spouses, parents and close relatives have become victims of medical over utilization con artistry that's sinful and then you realize America's health delivery system has hit an almost unbelievable low point due to its economic dilemma.

"Bottomry" began in medieval times. By the late 17th century intelligent men gathered at Edward Lloyd's coffee shop in London. Together variably large and larger sums of money were put at risk in a pool to protect ships and their owners from storms and piracy. Merchants, ship owners and mercantilists that produced then exported and delivered products, in exchange for solid currency or its equivalent, had spread the risk. Individuals, companies and corporations were saved from huge losses capable of bankrupting their operations.

Malpractice insurance has been carried by hospitals to prevent unrealistic jury awards from closing them down. The insurance lobby over decades since WW II has become the most powerful lobby in the nation, probably in all 50 states. This had best be kept in mind in case you expect quick sociological change. The reason your insurance cost has doubled or tripled what it should is because so many insured show disrespect for the principle that began the concept of insurance in the first place. Actuaries have continued to adjust rates from calculations and predictions of irrational expectancy, bad faith actions, greed, ignorance or just many folk that don't care about anyone else. This has meant the rates for the honest insured go up.

A "technological revolution" of the late 20th century has caused hospitals to become loaded with expensive hi-tech equipment. It has also fostered monopolistic practices. Major insurance companies have by 2000 begun to admit to the impact of drug costs as well. The pharmaceutical cartel has continued to excessively charge distributors, hospitals, community pharmacy outlets, patients and/or their insurance carriers whenever a new patented medicine becomes a marketing success. Hospital pharmacies have been stocked with high priced drugs. Striving for monopoly began with the Industrial Revolution. Subsequently forgotten, "Laissez faire" proved the ruination of mercantilism. Deregulation was touted again as the way to promote competition and, as a result, lower costs but oh, my, just look at what has happened since the nineteen eighties!

Do you have confidence General Electric, by providing hospitals with very expensive and sophisticated machines, will give us the necessary answers to diseases thus far unexplained?

People expect that cures for unexplained diseases are forthcoming because of the sophisticated looks of this expensive equipment. With completion of the human genome project people believe gene transplants are just around the corner. If gene transplant procedures become available in major city medical centers is there going to be anyone who can afford it? But, don't worry because the gene for cystic fibrosis on chromosome 7 was identified nearly 20 years ago and there is no gene transplant correction as yet for this most common mutation that includes 1 per 2400 white and 1 per 17,000 black births? When and if it ever is done who exactly is going to pay for the "six million dollar child?" No one seems willing to admit there are limits to everything?

A real doctor measures a patient's progress by questioning and observing the patient! Because calcifications appears less, clots or masses measure smaller, or a mentally ill schizophrenic takes up a little more radioactive glucose in his or her frontal lobes, in comparison to three months ago, it doesn't mean the patient feels better or that quality of life and daily living are improving. Nowadays a physician asks, "How do you feel?" The patient responds out of misery, "How many scans are you going to take?" "I don't feel any better no matter what the scan shows!" Doctors now tend to ignore what the patient says. They lecture by showing an audience scans and how the scans have improved. The gamma knife clearly takes away a brain metastases. It's no longer visible. Does the patient feel better? No! The scan however looks 100% better!

A good medical history is still the most important. Of course scanners help. The x-ray slices of computerized tomography (the CT scan) identify calcifications in the choroid as the mysterious cause of a rare patient's visual loss. Magnetic resonance imaging (MRI) generating its pictures from the magnetic twisting and relaxing of the nucleus of the hydrogen atom (proton) gives a very sharp demarcation between fat, CH-CH=CH-CH, etc; and water HHO to easily perceive normal brain tissue or a blood clot or some other mass. There's a useful single photon tomogram and also a two photon, positron emission scan called PET that measures radio active glucose uptake by the brain's nerve cells.

Everyone looks to the hospital and its gadgets. Yet being an anatomist or a radiologist doesn't make anyone the most helpful or kind practicing physician. The challenge to interpret disease still requires an emphasis on fundamentals. Serendipity is very important but physician's minds now are mostly prepared to look for money! Lemons and oranges prevent scurvy says a 18th century naval surgeon. Quinine benefits malaria 200 years before anyone knows some mosquito causes it. Milkmaids with cowpox never get small pox, the worst scourge of mankind, thus vaccination prevents small pox says an English physician in 1801. A 19th century Austrian physician says wash your hands! Quinine regulates an irregular heartbeat as shown by a Dutch sea captain in 1914. A fungus in a petri dish destroys bacteria says a Scottish bacteriologist in 1928! A dye antagonizes bacteria says a German chemist in 1932. Amantadine for the "flu" helps a Parkinsonian patient says a Harvard neurology professor about 1970! All this without any of those hi-tech gadgets! What do you say to that General Electric? Have any of your machines done anything like that? Go fly your airplane engines! Give the hospitals a break!

And there is no sense being hospitalized unless it is absolutely necessary. There's no sense dwelling over some disease. In the mail comes a web site opportunity, a comprehensive library with up to date coverage of 101 common disorders and conditions. Every "worry on the list" is familiar. Each deserves comment based on the fundamentals of common sense to allay patient anxiety. Should you subscribe to this? What is your purpose? Are you going to advise your doctor what bad condition you believe you must have, so maybe you can be "hospitalized?" Good physicians resist this type thing. No, you don't have Lyme disease! No, you don't have sarcoidosis! And, getting gastroenteritis on a cruise ship is no different than getting it on shore! Regardless, there is a growing "do it yourself trend" countrywide. People use the Internet to interpret the meaning of their symptoms. We enter the 21st century to the tune of "backwardness" relying too much on hi-tech instrumentation. You cannot learn the practice of medicine through gadgets. Good medicine could be practiced on perhaps five percent of the gross domestic product rather than 15 percent, if people thought a minute and stopped outsmarting themselves. The Canadian Plan, corrupted as it is by corporate America with especially too many scanners, still hangs in to manage pretty well on about 9 percent.

What about the American Medical Association generating millions of dollars selling biographies of certain select physicians? Do they search through medical centers and major hospital staffs to find the physician and take a vote? Is it the doctor that orders all the tests almost all the time? Does the pharmaceutical industry provide funding for professors of medical centers, the same as paying sops to say favorable things about certain products to advance sales? Does the drug cartel have some say about all this?

What about Alzheimer's disease programs in hospitals? Are patients put into these programs when loss of faculties occurs as a result of a risk of surgery? How many of the inmates of the program are confirmed by brain biopsy diagnosis? If the biopsy reveals the plaques and neurofibrillary tangles and the amyloid protein consistent with what Alzheimer observed over 100 years ago is this the result of many varied conditions or just one disease? This is still a reasonable question. It always comes up when television ads show men and women in white lab coats ("scientists associated with a pharmaceutical firm") posed like a flock of geese in "V formation," promising a "vaccine for Alzheimer's disease." Why do we have to be exposed to such "hot air full of false promises?" (Too bad we didn't have television in 1940 when sulfanilamide the red azo dye derivative, initiating a real new era in medicine, was 20 cents a tablet in the US and just 4 cents in Mexico! That was something tangible, and certain people really (!) benefited. That's a television ad that I would applaud.)

The reason hospitals are just like other employers of people has been financial considerations so overwhelming it forces this obvious lack of "hospitality" on all of us nationwide. Collectively society must come to its' senses and begin to redefine the overall value of the hospital. Unless good will begins to reemerge and there's a remarkable improvement in medical political strategies, the United States will begin to fail substantially as a civilization during the 21st century. Hospitals must serve all the masses, not just the rich and insured. Why doesn't the US Congress see this?

Think bout "Mother Goose" and all you can learn from such a source. And there's one particular nursery rhyme that may apply: Humpty Dumpty sat high on a wall. Humpty Dumpty had a great fall. All the king's horses and all the king's men couldn't put Humpty Dumpty (the US) together again!

Hillary Rodham Clinton, senator for the state of New York as first lady wrote a book: "It Takes a Village." The physicians and the hospital in that village better be good ones! No one sick or injured should be turned away.

CHAPTER IV

BRAINS AND BRAWN

Anabolic Steroids, East versus West and 'Politics with Muscle.'

"What's the use of prohibition, you'll produce the same condition
Crazy rhythm, I'm going crazy too."

"Folker, please tell me you're kidding; you know teenagers in Germany taking beta guanidino propionic acid?" "It is crazy, but it's true," Folker replied. "You know, this really interests me. Beta guanidino propionic acid is the "trip to Mars stuff," to help maintain enough strength so you can still move around when you get there!

Believe it or not I've been a "weight lifter" since age 15. All through medical school and internship, with little sleep, no vitamin supplements by the way, and devoting maybe six hours a week for heavy lifting; well, I competed in key meets. Qualifying for the Olympic Games was out of the question, however, I snatched 270 and clean and jerked 330 pounds; finished first in 30 regional AAU meets in the 181 to 198 pound class most years from 1952 to 1962. The idea was do it on your own stuff. In those days there were enough vitamins in just plain good food. That's how I looked at it, but some of my competitors took alfalfa extracts, drank an extra quart of milk a day, or, ate pounds of horse meat, purchased at Scotty's Pony Market in Oakland. Actually I tried a few horse meat sandwiches. Meat from the horse, those large lean pieces, was about 40 cents a pound. But those chewy little blood vessels in that kind of meat proved too much for me. It was soon back to beef! Dr. Lucas, quite famous, of the UCSF orthopedic department, wanted to give me a spinal tap to record cerebral spinal fluid pressures during a lift." "Did you do it" Folker asked? "No, no, no," I told him, "I can't do that! Members of the orthopedic department were very "curious researchers," but they overlooked my concern about one whopper of a post spinal headache, from loss of cerebral spinal fluid, and, a bent needle!"

Professor Folker Hanefeld of Gottingen Germany and I were part of the delegation at the International Symposium on multiple sclerosis held in Budapest Hungary, during September 1994. We befriended each other since, in his presentation, he really surprised me with the very mention of beta guanidino propionic acid. He used it for correcting documented low levels of creatine in central nervous system white matter.

As a result Professor Hanefeld was delighted with my "public relations proposal." Returning to California I telephoned Dr. Kenneth Baldwin, researcher in the field of muscle physiology at UC Irvine. His work was backed by a research grant from the National Aeronautics and Space Administration (NASA). Among other things Dr. Baldwin had been giving beta guanidino propionic acid to rats as a method of "depleting phosphate energized creatine" in their skeletal muscles. It was as though the rats had engaged in a workout when, in fact, the rats hadn't performed any muscular activity beyond their usual routine. Such investigations were of the utmost importance for planning a manned trip to Mars, meaning about a year in space round trip!

I'm not the one to give a good answer why someone actually wants to go to Mars. Speaking of being fearful of change. During 1994, Chinese businessmen in Hong Kong are happy with just a prospect for success involving a trip to Vancouver, Western Canada. Now they go back and forth regularly, and have done so for several years. I do not anticipate too much back and forth to Mars but it is not within my province to say. Some are very anxious to get going.

Where muscle power in space is concerned Soviet cosmonauts, as the first to go aloft for long periods in their space station, sometimes could not even stand up returning from zero gravity back to Earth. On the more positive side a physician cosmonaut, Valery Polyakov, set the record for weightless space flight of 437 days, returning to Kazakhstan in 1995 walking away so they said under his own power! Meeting veteran astronaut, Senator John Glenn in Washington DC, Polyakov asked Glenn if he'd like to fly to Mars, and Glenn replied, "With 'you' Valery, anytime!" One logically concludes that the Soviet cosmonaut physician hero managed his stay in space so unexpectedly well on something more than "resistance exercises in zero gravitational forces." Is he getting a boost from a special recipe to keep his skeletal muscles fit and with just a little bone loss?

Why the approval for what ever is necessary for travelers in space yet such vehement disapproval of athletes like shot put champion Randy Barnes? Many years ago he and hundreds of other world class athletes discover something more than a high calorie, high protein diet was absolutely necessary in order to train hard enough and long enough to put a sixteen pound shot 75 feet 7 inches, the all time world record? Isn't going to Mars a kind of "sporting event?" Isn't there going to be a spectacular crowd of spectators to observe those who dare to take off and hopefully return from the red planet fourth from the sun? And in terms of giving spectators what they yearn for, thinking of professional sports in particular, aren't anabolic steroids being used now for decades by so many athletes competing in football, wrestling, baseball, tennis and boxing?

For skeletal muscles to serve you best for your competitive task at hand, you must use those muscles in a strategic manner. "Creatine" is in blood, brain and "muscles." It is synthesized from two dietary essential amino acids, arginine and methionine plus an amino acid synthesized in the human body, glycine. If you take extra creatine in your diet, is that going to give you more muscle power? No! The creatine must be synthesized! Is taking more glycine, arginine and methionine going to give you more muscle? No! But, if you take extra amounts of these three amino acids, you can find out whether you are able to train harder and for longer periods, with improved recuperation, brought about by "accelerating the synthesis of more skeletal muscle." You might increase your competitive performance more than you would normally expect within a certain investment of training time. I don't know for sure. Glycine being very much involved in transmission of nerve impulse, is taking an extra amount of glycine going to speed up your reflexes? No!

With the brain and the endocrine system and the skeletal muscle system to consider, there has been altogether too much involved to understand. Before divorces became common, for anyone engaged to be married, everything associated with all the anticipation, excitement, enthusiasm and happiness speeded things up! There was "more energy" to expend. When on the other hand you got divorced, with the loss of trust, disappointments, (trying to cook for yourself!), and the spite and legal maneuvering, you have "less energy." There are stories of great competitive athletes quitting competition forever after a divorce! The human body is a very complex biochemical system that involves maybe twice as many enzymatic reactions from 35000 gene expressions!

Does taking beta guanidino propionic acid, since it "depletes skeletal muscle 'creatine' energized with phosphate," foster some production of more creatine? That could be the case! We ought to ask what some of those teenagers in Gottingen Germany are saying about it? Is beta guanidino propionic acid "all" they are taking? Are these short cut oriented teenagers also taking anabolic steroids? Are they able to afford growth hormone injections? Are they taking erythropoietin or Epoetin? Isn't it a fact there are young athletes nowadays willing to take anything that enables a way to train full time, to achieve the sports performance they dream about? And what is the sense if you are not naturally a great athlete in the first place? Put another way, if you have an IQ of 100 and there's a pill taken for a couple years to raise your IQ to 120 (no such medicine or herb exists, however, remember that!), then what's the sense if what you are dreaming about requires an IQ of 140?

Are those planning to travel to Mars going be to given something besides all those "energizing breakfast cereals," so they may accomplish their task, given every single possible advantage? Of course, otherwise why would NASA sponsor medical research on skeletal muscle? What's better, putting the shot 75 feet, or, going to Mars? It depends upon what certain individuals would like to accomplish. Both goals are reasonable for those motivated to advance in either direction. It's fun to watch anyone perform a feat.

Gifted comedian-tragedian writer, Cyrano de Bergerac expresses his feelings, in his "Voyages to the Moon" published in 1655, "There are those who yearn to explore the Earth's atmosphere and look back at our Earth with islands of land surrounded by water, like those brave explorers of the sea tell us." Likewise, there are those who yearn to perform athletic feats without leaving our Earth, not satisfied with a sixty foot toss of a 16 pound steel ball, something Parry O'Brien did on his own natural ability. They wish to toss it further, or as far as humanly possible. The record books show athletic records have increased dramatically over the past fifty years. Those cheering on their favorite performers expect now these sensational performances. There is no remaining enthusiasm today for watching nineteen fifties records. However, there is enthusiasm for witnessing performances of athletes who train to compete in various events that are now full time occupations. On September 14, 2002 sprinter Tim Montgomery exploded for the crowd in Paris France, breaking Maurice Green's world record of 9.79 in the one hundred meter dash with a time of 9.78 seconds! A number of financial rewards for Tim Montgomery's remarkable feat totaled half a million dollars US! What does that tell you?

NASA may employ physicians, as well as researchers with a Ph.D., to work on "putting a man on Mars experiments." Where sports on Earth are concerned physicians participate to instill fears and try to make athletes out like criminals who are dedicated to doing their best in competition! Athletes as a result play the game of not getting caught for doing what the athlete must do to compete successfully, especially at the highest level, and thus every legal tactic through courtrooms must be employed to keep certain athletes in the competition.

Valery Polyakov, who set the world record for weightless space flight, was first and foremost a Soviet physician. Interestingly, about 1950 the Soviets initiated an experiment that had to do with increasing the ability for human skeletal muscle to perform lifts, not for endurance in space, but for competitive sporting events. That experiment began with another Soviet physician by the name of Arcadi Vorobiev, champion for lifting a barbell from the floor to overhead.

Hormone research prior to World War II in the United States and Europe focused on adrenal cortical tissue, 85 percent of the hormones in such tissue being anti-inflammatory and catabolic (break down not build up skeletal muscle), with assigned names cortisone and hydrocortisone. Experiments by the early nineteen fifties in the United States and in the Soviet Union involved sex hormones as well as their precursors. They were "anabolic, nitrogen retaining," for building and rebuilding muscle and tendon tissue. In addition to adrenal cortical activity there was activity to see what could be achieved making more anabolic Testosterone available in the male, and anabolic Estrogen in the female.

In truth both the US and the Soviets succeeded with their experiments! Norethynodrel-Mestranol, the "Pill," was released in the US in 1956. It consisted of a combination, not one but "two 'anabolic steroids'." Within ten years seven million women were taking such oral contraceptives to prevent pregnancy by inhibition of ovulation by interference with hypothalamic-pituitary mechanisms! The Soviets began their experiments with the intent of improving all kinds of athletic performances. Physicians and coaches administered to their selected best athletic prospects amounts of male hormone Testosterone to discover these athletes were able then to train longer and harder and, of course, really improve!

In 1956, at the Melbourne Australia Olympic Games, physician Arcadi Vorobiev, weighing little more than 190 pounds, astounded the weightlifting world with an Olympic styled press of 325 pounds! The lift was performed very quickly, and so astoundingly it was ruled acceptable by the judges. By rules in place it didn't "really qualify as a press." Astonishing to watch, the feat baffled judges and coaches as well as the audience. It also amazed US lifter, David Sheppard, probably the most "naturally gifted of all Olympic Games styled lifters."

Dave Sheppard won the silver medal on just the hormones God gave him. He suffered a fractured arm trying for the gold with then a total of the three lifts exceeding Vorobiev's total. He gave his all in the third event, the clean and jerk, with enough poundage to overtake Arcadi, but missed to sustain the injury. Tommy Kono and Paul Anderson, the Dixie derrick, Paul ill from "flu" or "food poisoning," losing 40 pounds (!), just managed to edge Silvetti of Argentina. Both won gold medals for the US but, from 1956 onward, the Soviets and East Bloc countries developed athletic training programs with intentions of leaving all other world class competitors behind.

Preventing pregnancy with hormone prescriptions was important to the West. The prestige of winning world championships in athletics was important to the East. In the US, no one by 1956 was able to understand how Russian athletes were able to train so heavily for such long periods, every week for 52 weeks a year! Bob Hoffman of York, weight lifting coach for the US exclaimed, "If you want to beat the Russians, you have to train like the Russians!" The trouble was, "it took an athlete with God given 'designer genes' to train heavily as much as ten hours per week," whereas the Soviet steroid programs enabled their athletes to train "three times that long, or, '30 hours' per week (!)," and keep bouncing back for more!

From a legal point of view considering "intent," researchers in the US were in a better position to predict therapeutic prevention of pregnancy, taking two sex hormones albeit weaker anabolic hormones than Testosterone, than were the Soviet experimenters. There had to be very little confidence that giving extra Testosterone to East Bloc athletes particularly those already quite fully developed would help them in any way. In fact physicians in the US scoffed at the idea! The truth as it turned out just taking the Testosterone failed to improve athletic performances. It was not a case of making progress without more exercise. The administered Testosterone enabled them to train longer and harder than anyone dreamed possible. All that was left to do was arrange time periods for Soviet and East Bloc athletes to train long enough, to make use of (use up) the extra hormone prescriptions. It paved the way for the athlete to train with enthusiasm 30 hours per week and become no longer the amateur but a "full time jock."

The last "amateur" Olympic Games was held in London, England in 1948. After the Helsinki, Finland Olympic Games in 1952 US Olympic weightlifting coach, Bob Hoffman, wondered how the Russians were training by showing so much more improvement than anticipated. It wasn't just a matter of determination, they were really getting better! Stalin was very much alive in 1952 along with Malenkov, Bulganin and Krushchev. Had shot putters, discus throwers, javelin and hammer throwers or the Hoffman team of US weight lifters accepted an invitation to visit the Soviet Union in 1952, they might have gotten too scared to perform. It was three years after Stalin's death during 1956 the US State Department gave approval for American weight lifters, Tommy Kono, David Sheppard and, Paul Anderson to go to Moscow. They were welcomed and really wowed a packed audience in Russia's major city.

Dictator Joseph Stalin, the "man of steel" died in 1953, the same year the Soviets acquired the Hydrogen bomb. These were very difficult times. Four years earlier the Soviets, by 1949, perfected an Atomic bomb as no surprise. The Soviets showed they were as good in science as the US. After all they had scientist, Lev Davidovich Landau, the math prodigy who worked with Niels Bohr in 1934 and became head of the USSR Academy of Science in 1937. (Landau won the Nobel Prize in physics in 1962 for his accomplishments in the field of super fluidity.)

It was not until March 1958 that Nikita Krushchev successfully struggled to become leader of the Soviet Union. Krushchev, like Trotsky, overwhelmingly embraced communism. Krushchev proved very different from Stalin. Stalin, the dictator, was steadfastly focused only on the future welfare and security of the Soviet Union. Stalin, who had the West so frightened was by hindsight never a threat to the United States. It was Krushchev, unlike Stalin, who began strutting his stuff to espouse communism worldwide. That was what Trotsky did and logically why Stalin ordered Trotsky assassinated in Mexico City by 1940. From his poor judgments of WW I leading up to September 1, 1939, Stalin was probably convinced Trotsky "had lost his mind." Krushchev had something, however, beyond Trotsky's wildest dreams: inter-continental missiles, atomic warheads, and hydrogen bombs to back him up! It was this very problem that caused staggering worldwide tensions, and finally, the worst crisis the US ever faced up to 2003, namely the "Cuban missile crisis of 1962," the word "crisis" being ameliorative.

Deceptively as a superficial gesture Krushchev encouraged world class athletic competitions between the United States and Russia. Such an encouragement along with much lip service lulled some in the US to think of Krushchev as sometimes quite a jovial and very congenial world leader. (In actuality he was a much greater threat to the US than Saddam Hussein ever was (except for all the problems involving Middle East "oil"), or anyone else. Stalin was feared and also tactically misunderstood so much top-secret information never made public. Stalin was grateful for America's help tilting the balance to make the winning of World War I possible. Stalin was released from the gulag as a result! Also, by winning WW I, the treaty of Brest-Litovsk, negotiated by Trotsky, was nullified. This enabled the Soviet Union to get back the mineral rich Ukraine! Stalin was also grateful for America's help during the Battle of Britain, and for lend- lease packages prior to America entering WW II. In Battles of Britain from Nazi invasion, some 107,000 British pilots, 84,000 American pilots and 42,200 Soviet pilots were killed in a combined force that included volunteers from Australia, Canada, India, Rhodesia, South Africa, Belgium, Czechoslovakia, Denmark, France, Greece, Netherlands, Norway and Poland. The Battle of Britain represented the monumental supreme cooperative and successful effort to hold off Germany's world's most powerful air force from weakening England, enabling then a relatively easy German occupation. Furthermore, it was such an outstanding combined effort. It was the second front that gave Hitler more than his unbelievably powerful army could handle, albeit not by much. It was only with the help of the Soviet Union that enabled the allied forces to win WW II. And it was America, Britain, Australian and many other forces that saved the Soviet Union! Krushchev somewhat surprisingly continually bashed Stalin in the late fifties, knowing of no better way to make him self look good especially to those in countries bordering the Soviet Union.) No matter what, world class athletes from the US and Russia were much happier with now the prospect of such great competition, and also the comradeship. The secrets of the East Bloc's phenomenal sports program were graciously related to those of the West Bloc, one super athlete to another. Just like the great success with the birth control pill, the Russians couldn't wait to tell the US athletes what they were taking to help them build more muscle. It was the athletes both East and West that wanted an even playing field and may the best man win.

By the fall of 1958 the mystery of what was taking place in the realm of world championship athletics was revealed. Russian field athletes shared their "Dianabol secret" with competing American athletes. The oral anabolic steroid named "Dianabol" became available in the United States that year. The little blue tablets were now beginning to "work their miracle." US competitors were making gains, simply by being able to train longer and harder. In truth it was quite amazing. But, in order to put in the extra training demanded by the use of anabolic steroids, various businesses like the Bank of America allotted time off to a very top athletic prospect that happened to be one of their employees. In short, American businesses became sponsors. It was, "Let's all rise to the occasion, compete with the East Bloc and 'beat' the Russians." For athletics it was a great time. It became "East versus West."

With close friends and many acquaintances in track and field, world class USC shot putter, Davie Davis, second to Parry O'Brien, first to break the 60 foot barrier on his own natural stuff, paid me a visit during internship at Harbor General-UCLA Hospital in Torrance California. Davie asked what I thought about his taking Dianabol (methandrostenolone). Looking at Davie weighing a solid 255 pounds, I said, "I'm using 'Dianabol' on the 'female' orthopedic right now. It's to speed up healing of broken femurs in elderly ladies! I don't understand how in the world it would be useful for someone, already fully developed, especially a muscular hulk like you!" Davie Davis replied, " 'Doc,' I just got back from a world meet. The Russians told me they're taking it. I'm taking some for just two months, training much harder and my shot went from 61 feet to 63 feet five inches! That conversation took place the very day a USC shot putter taught a doctor something and the doctor (me) never saw Davie Davis looking quite so pleased. He had broken through his frustrating, "sticking point." The anabolic steroids were letting him train harder and longer. Other famous jocks were also beginning to get the idea!

By the Rome Olympic Games of 1960 the secret for training longer and harder was known by virtually all the top athletes of the West, but it was kept within the policy makers of international sports since many if not all were simply convinced there was nothing to it. Top level athletes of the West as of 1958 were following East Bloc established practices using anabolic steroids like Dianabol. Both sides were enthusiastically preparing for the Rome Games. US athletes along with essentially all the top qualifiers of the West Bloc were aiming for the Olympic trials and looking ahead at last to an even playing field. The East Bloc with its' previous Testosterone experience had the benefit, however, of one great head start! By the time of the Rome Games, the furthest shot put by anyone not taking anabolic steroids was 60 feet ten inches by Charles Robert Butt, son of Edward Butt, one time chairman of the University of Southern California's medical center's pathology department.   The furthest discus throw by anyone not using exogenous anabolic steroids was 201 feet by Bob Humphreys, who years later used his great all around talent as a place kicker in pro football. Soon, however, 60foot shot puts and 200foot discus throws proved not enough to please spectator buffs involved in world class sport pageants.

Robert Burns Aird, M.D., neurological surgeon from Harvard, turned neurologist and who after WW II founded the UCSF neurology department introduced me to virtually every famous neurologist in the world. If not at UCSF, introductions took place during travels to meetings and congresses, from the nineteen seventies to the nineteen nineties. In 1985, at Hamburg, Germany, Bob introduced me to fellow neurologist Roger Bannister. Sir Roger Bannister, British physician, was the first to succeed running a carefully measured mile in less than four minutes, a feat champion runners before him thought perhaps not possible. (That great record occurred on May 6, 1954, a time of 3 minutes 59.4 seconds!) In our discussion Roger, like myself, wished anabolic steroids had never worked; that they had made no difference. In response to the obvious and to anyone curious, "extra anabolic steroids have made a big difference," Roger was quoted in newspapers worldwide saying, "Athletes using anabolic steroids were engaged in doing something "very, very wrong." His viewpoint was understandable. (What about the "sport" of putting a man on Mars?)

"Talk about terribly unfair!" Those were his very words during a personal conversation with my friend, Los Angeles barrister David Matlin, leading United States official for Olympic weight lifting at the 1976 Olympics in Montreal Canada. He said, "Phil Grippaldi's 198 pound class bronze medal was taken away from Phil and awarded to the fourth place finisher of the East Bloc, who wasn't tested at all! "He wasn't given a urine test for anabolic steroids 'everybody knew he was taking'!" Grippaldi was singled out and humiliated as if to imply all other weight lift competitors were innocent! Grippaldi was suspended from competition for a year! By testing only "every 'sixth' athlete," politicians and promoters of the Games "covered up what had been going for the previous 18 years!" Every weight lifter and field athlete knew none of them could have even qualified for the Olympic trials without taking anabolic steroids. The anabolic steroids enabled the athletes to spend those needed extra hours of training made possible by accelerated muscle rebuilding and much, much quicker recovery from heavy intensive workouts.

No wonder attorney David Matlin was upset. By utilizing a policy that tested only one of every six competitors a form of "Russian roulette" was invoked. In the original form using a revolver, if you lost you were dead. In this modified form, for athletes dedicated to world sporting events, if you lost through a urine test you just wished you were dead! It became all the more agonizing since there was an "awareness of 'preferential' treatment!" How was it certain star competitors, favorably mentioned repeatedly in the news media, and therefore "best able to draw attendance," (Box office appeal) somehow escaped testing? Was it because each one represented a drawing card for promoters, or, was it just the luck of the draw? Wasn't it "sports politics?"

Within the political framework of international sports, a new kind of competition emerged to pit East versus West. Ironically this competition also had a West versus West component. Lab buffs of the United States and Germany were vying for who was to become the "undisputed champion of urine testing!" This policy became another challenge for all world class athletes.

With all the worldwide newspaper publicity, people were coming out of the woodwork for some kind of "credit." One doctor's lamentation he was so sorry that he helped "create Dianabol." A champion "power lifter" (not an Olympic Games event) that involves bench press, squat and dead lift and with a physique like a Greek statue became a candidate for coronary by-pass surgery. Anabolic steroids were the focus of blame. What else was responsible? Family history? Had anybody bothered to ask? Overlooked was his confession. He admitted to ingesting food, measuring 11,000 calories per day (!), including 30 eggs daily (!), along with three pounds of meat! (*Gene chips for sequential testing were not then available.)

Even a gorilla knew better than to eat 30 eggs a day! In fact the book published in 1978, "All about Gorillas," by David. P. Willoughby, revealed gorillas typically ate "just six eggs each morning," along with powdered milk, sugar, codfish liver oil, vitamins and a gallon of water. About 2:00 PM gorillas opted for bunches of celery, beets, carrots, one scallion, three pounds of string beans, one and one half pounds of chopped, well cooked, horse meat, 12 oranges, 20 apples, six pounds of bananas, and a pound of grapes. Along with that they ate various other fruits in season like peaches, pears, cherries, cantaloupes and pineapples. Well, if all this exceeded 11,000 calories, at least the gorillas ate 24 fewer eggs per day than the troubled bodybuilder. (Note: Nevertheless, one should not jump to a "conclusion" eating 30 eggs daily automatically leads to occlusion of one's coronary arteries. There is more to it than that but, psychologically, I wouldn't go that far no matter how much I appreciate chickens.)

Willoughby told me it was unfair to compare a man with a gorilla, simply because no matter what humans ate, how long or hard they trained or what anabolic steroids they took, a human could never match especially the grip of a gorilla. Amusingly gorillas have been evaluated as being physically worth more than the human body builder. (Arnold Schwarzeneggar, the movie star, being a remarkable exception) Chicago's Lincoln Park Zoos' Francis X. Bushman was given a value of $100,000 at age 18 back in 1946! Many other famous gorillas like King Tut, Albert, and Massa, for example like Bushman, were of great value and naturally much stronger than any man.

By 1970 cardiologists, sports physicians, and various other interested persons, became convinced they were experts on nutrition. This was a result of intense committee meetings that simply overlooked gaps in our knowledge regarding nutrition that still remain today. One certain diet was best for heavy weight lifts, puts and weight throws, another diet for sprints, and something different for distance running, and of course special diets to prevent blood vessels from becoming obstructed. The fear of eggs had hit its' zenith. Butter had taken a hit as well. Fear was promulgated, and connected to the imagination of both physicians and lay persons over the use of anabolic steroids!

Many athletes wondered what the fuss was all about having used anabolic steroids regularly since 1958, feeling fine, performing in their chosen sport better than ever and, looking terrific. There of course were certain athletes that fell prey to by then well established forms of contemporary drug abuse, beginning with marijuana and going on from there. They suffered like others involved with such abuses that had no interest in athletics whatever. And yet anabolic steroids were repeatedly singled out.

Physicians were not sought out as those who knew much about anabolic steroids. Their significance for world class athletes preparing for world competition hadn't engaged the interest of most doctors. However there were physicians, particularly internists with special interest in endocrinology prescribing anabolic steroids to athletes and following their progress carefully. There was one Sacramento internist who prescribed the right amount of anabolic hormone for his son whom I saw training frequently at the downtown Sacramento California YMCA. His son was a very polite young fellow, very strong with an impressive physique. He showed not a sign of any side effects. "International sports policies," however, took on such proportions even physicians interested became afraid to stay involved. Physicians with experience in this area were intimidated and driven out. To those knowledgeable about anabolic steroids being used East versus West for years the policy made no medical sense at all.

It became easier to prescribe morphine for pain than prescribe anabolic steroids to help an athlete train heavier and longer. There was a federal drug policy that placed a physician under suspicion that he might be using morphine himself in conjunction with administering morphine to patients to ease the horrific pains of terminal cancer. There was more reasonable suspicion for morphine being taken by a prescribing physician, than for some doctor to take anabolic steroids because he prescribed them. Still there were physicians fearful of taking charge of their own practicing situation.

Pompous attitudes of certain physicians very involved in sports caused accomplished athletes looking in their direction to sense they were looking at the wrong end of a horse! To wit, one physician, who on his best day couldn't throw a discus 40 feet nevertheless felt qualified to explain what was involved in this event to Jay Sylvester who performed a discus throw of 225 feet! It was considered outrageous, at least irreverent, for an athlete like Sylvester to offer any opinion about how he accomplished what he did to "some doctor sir, your lordship," heading up a prestigious national and international sports committee.

Dangers associated with taking anabolic steroids became an international obsession and never mind attempts to gain clinical experience privately by asking athletes who had taken anabolic steroids for years about any significant side effects. Unlikely side effects were targeted and, as with all prescription drugs, of course there were some! In 1974 at any rate a "Ban" was formally instituted. "This Ban made anabolic steroids 'illegal' for athletes." For 22 years anabolic steroids had been "legal" for East Bloc competitors! For 16 years, from 1958 to 1974, they had been "legal" for competitors of the US and the West! Clearly when anything perfectly legal was to become suddenly illegal, problems of all kinds were bound to arise. It was totally a magisterial decision. Problems did arise, to put it mildly!

The "Ban" caused interpersonal difficulties, between competitors and coaches in world sports. There was also a significant political misfortune associated with "the timing of the Anabolic Steroid Ban of 1974". It was the very year Leonid Brezhnev at last ousted Khrushchev (!), and by doing so established "détente" between the Soviet Union and the United States! Politically ignoring an opportunity for improving relations in world's sports, the "Ban" was instead accelerated into high gear creating "preferential treatment and needless stressful difficulties in association with the 1976 Montreal Olympic Games and continuing right on into 1977.

In 1977 with the Ban in full force, Brezhnev became president of the Soviet Union, and let it be known to everyone in the world of his immense pleasure Moscow had been selected for the 1980 summer Olympic Games! Athletes representing the United States were really looking forward to the Olympics to be held in Moscow. Deep inside there was some kind of confident feeling, "at least a sincere hope that the KGB would assure all urine tests were reported normal, to sensibly restore East versus West competition fair and square." After all, those Olympic Games in Rome 1960, in Tokyo 1964, in Mexico City 1968 as well as Munich 1972 were all "anabolic steroid 'legal' Olympic Games." Steroids were legal before 1974!"

America's foreign policy advisors blinded by the idea of "fighting communism," to an extent of being unwilling to ease up on athletic competition for the sake of improving international relationships, declared the US would not participate in the Moscow Olympic Games! Very troublesome uprisings in Afghanistan engaging the Soviet Union were given as the reason America's top athletes would not be permitted to compete in Moscow. Going still further, of all things, the planned sale to Russia of "our excess wheat in America's mid west" was not to take place either! Brezhnev, disappointed and unable to persuade America to change its' mind, but not lacking a sense of humor, determined to make sure other West Bloc countries competed. He made West German newspaper headlines: "Come See Us before We Come See You!" West Germany understandably showed up in Moscow and competed in the '80 Games! In the US, political tensions seemed greater over anabolic steroid usage among athletes than over the escalating war in Afghanistan, which also became our business.

No one knew more about the value of international sports relationships than US shot put star, Al Feuerbach. In the nineteen seventies Al Feuerbach held the world record for the shot put at 71 feet 7 inches. A great competitor in Olympic styled weightlifting as well, Al Feuerbach was a big man, except in comparison to his competitors that were much bigger. He became the world record holder by using anabolic steroids in a professional manner and by training very, very hard. This was made very clear on sports pages of US newspapers coast to coast. He also emphasized the healthy relationship of East versus West Bloc sports competition. Al had precedents, logic and reason on his side as well as facts, facts that judges in courtrooms absolutely yearn for, yet nothing proved sufficient to argue successfully against the sports politicians that created the "Ban, of 1974."

Overlooking logic and reason along with the US, British newspaper releases chastised and humiliated Britain's very best field athletes. Their champion in the shot put was called "a cheat and a fool!" Such criticism was meant for all their other athletes of the field meaning those trained in the hammer, discus and javelin. It stirred up heated conversation in the pubs.

On December 16, 1983, William E. Simon, president of the United States Olympic committee answered my letter of a couple weeks previous. He answered it in a very polite way but had obviously been "personally persuaded of the great dangers of anabolic steroids for athletes." In paragraph five he stated: "If, however, we (the US) are at a disadvantage because we "protect our 'athletes' health even that is a secondary matter to us." In other words his letter made very good sense based on what Mr. Simon "believed": It was better to stay healthy and lose in sports than win later on only to become ill from side effects of anabolic steroids. Only the shortsighted and obsessed were in disagreement with such a statement. Who, and where were all those athletes that had used anabolic steroids that damaged their health? Casually knowing Al Feuerbach, along with a number of star athletes who used anabolic steroids for years, particularly in the San Jose California area, it was difficult to either get to know or even learn of, or hear about, anyone ill from side effects of anabolic steroids! The few athletes in trouble everyone knew about were involved in various forms of contemporary drug abuse familiar to everyone. One weight lifter, very strong indeed, exhibited psychotic behavior attributable logically to amphetamines. His behavior proved upon personal observation indistinguishable from schizophrenia. He suffered delusions and was hearing voices and talking to this pillar in an auditorium. He certainly wasn't enraged in any way. He went up on the platform and calculatedly performed his lifts.

The "Ban on anabolic steroids" revealed some good sense judging in terms of clinical observations among East German female swimmers. During 1974 at an international swim meet held in Concord California, East German female swimmers performed, and how! Through the late Jack Kelly of Philadelphia I hoped to arrange a translator to inquire how the German female swimmers felt about their training program but in a very polite way. Jack Kelly had great interest in swimming, diving and, of course, "rowing" and was very well known for it. I had introduced him at the Comstock Club in Sacramento two days before the big swim meet and treated him to a tour of Sacramento. Jack especially wanted to see where swim phenomenon Mark Spitz trained under the auspices of his super swim coach Sherm Chavor. Much was discussed about sports, politics and a little about steroids and East Bloc female swimmers but an interview after the swim meet with the German girls, thinking Jack could arrange it, was not to be had. The lady swimmers all appeared happy and healthy. They seemed unconcerned or unaware of their male like musculature. Whatever anabolic program they were given it had created a virilizing effect due to blocked receptors for estrogen, or reduction in production of estrogen from testosterone, the physiologically documented normal pathway. Was winning worth it? Were no physicians involved in their intensive training program?

Concerning side effects of any medication, most medicines taken need to be metabolized and converted from a more lipid soluble to a more water soluble (or "polar") state for excretion by the kidneys. Usually everything goes well. Like the anti-psychotic medication, chlorpromazine better known as Thorazine, Dianabol sometimes causes an irritation and clogging of tiny bile passages in the liver. Thorazine can uncommonly cause jaundice via this mechanism as it is converted into chlorpromazine sulfoxide. The treatment of course: discontinue the drug (!) and allow biliary passges to get back to normal by eliminating the offending factor.

During 39 years of medical practice mainly neurology, 25 years of psychiatric medicine, along with some internal medicine I'm not personally aware, nor have been told of liver "malignancy," from Thorazine, one time most common prescription for schizophrenics. I'm likewise unaware that Dianabol, choice prescription many years with anabolic steroid programs, ever incited such a side effect. This personal experience is not meant to represent a completely reliable opinion.

One of my long time friends was Ken Zumwalt, for decades feature editor of the San Diego Union-Tribune. We wound up classmates at University of Maryland Extention in Frankfurt, Germany beginning in 1949. Ken was editor of "Stars and Stripes," America's overseas newspaper headquarters in Darmstadt, Germany. We kept in touch over many years and I really valued Ken's friendship. A newspaper article sent from Ken was by Lew Scarr of the San Diego Union-Tribune about steroids and the trials and tribulations of a San Diego orthopedist. The orthopedist in training amazingly had become a national collegiate heavyweight lifting champion. True to form Dianabol had been his favorite anabolic steroid. As a result of his intense training made possible only through Dianabol, budgeting the necessary time, he became qualified for the Olympic trials in 1960 and 1964! The article stated, however, he was prone to stasis of his liver bile passages from the Dianabol. He therefore was approached and agreed to become part of an experimental trial on another anabolic steroid known as Winthrol. Winthrol, however, also caused him to have abnormal liver function tests. These lab findings were interpreted as a forewarning of cholangiolytic jaundice (due to back up or clogging of bile passages). Wisely he quit taking any and all kinds of anabolic steroids. He simply accepted the fact he had no chance whatsoever (!), without those prescriptions, to train long and hard enough to consider "entering" Olympic trials, let alone qualify or have even a ghost of a chance of winning in international competition.

Regarding the difference anabolic steroid athletic programs have made in weight lifting a 20% increase in poundage has been accomplished within two years by devoting "three times as much time and effort into training." Olympic 198 pound (90 kg. weight class) champion of the 1948 London Olympic Games Norbert Schemansky performed a clean and jerk of 400 pounds (it was 399 pounds later on a scale but "400" in his mind) for a world and Olympic Games record. Had anabolic steroids been available enabling him to triple his training time he would have performed a clean and jerk of 500 pounds! A gain in body weight (skeletal muscle) of ten or more pounds would have placed him, however, in a heavier weight division.

Performing a shot put of 60 feet on natural ability might lead to 72 feet after two years on a properly prescribed steroid program. Dave Ashman, Southern California and Muscle Beach heavyweight class lifter, easily clean and jerked 440 pounds during the nineteen fifties. On an anabolic steroid program Ashman would have managed 540 pounds in that lift. However, in order to put in the time and effort to "use up his anabolic steroids," he wouldn't have been able to put in his regular hours as a Los Angeles policeman. Tragically Dave succumbed to illness unrelated to sports or steroids way before his time.

On testosterone and specialized anabolic steroids more than one Russian heavy weight lifter has threatened to clean and jerk 600 pounds (!), which on any program I believe is the limit of human possibility. Such a feat has much more meaning than a trip back and forth to Mars, if you are an athlete.

If bile passage clogging and jaundice did result from anabolic steroids would this mean, down the line, an athlete so affected would be (statistically) more likely to develop hepato cellular (liver), or bile duct malignancy? Some opine to this but my inclination is to doubt it. Hepatomas (liver tumors) are commonly associated with chronic alcoholism as well as hepatitis C. Conceivably two thirds of liver and related malignancy can be associated with either alcoholism or hepatitis C or the two in combination. If an athlete avoids alcohol and doesn't have hepatitis C, then simply using anabolic steroids while maintaining normal liver enzyme levels in the process raises little or no concern, by my clinical experience as regards liver disease later on. In terms of statistics, an Italian study published in 2001 suggests Estrogen, the predominant female anabolic hormone formed from Testosterone, "prevents colon and rectal cancer!" (Expect soon another journal article stating, no it doesn't!) Anabolic steroid sex hormones are believed by some to incite "this," prevent "that," but such claims arise from the utilization of too limited information to present reliable opinions. People have likened opinions to noses. Everybody has one! Many "opinions" have been published in medical literature. The lay public of course has expressed all kinds of opinions about everything. (Instead of airlines requesting a passport ask instead for an "opinion," and right away if you get one you know it's an American!) Sadly worthwhile opinions from random medical trials require decades to trickle down to practitioners for good judgment to be applied.

One of my patients had, confirmed at autopsy, a leiomyosarcoma of his bronchial tube with multiple brain metastases, indistinguishable from disseminated infection on CT scan. Oddly enough, treating the latter with four kinds of IV antibiotics (cost of antibiotic administration alone about $15,000), after each antibiotic the patient rallied from a semi comatose state to "up brushing his teeth and looking in the mirror!" His family thanked me four times for saving him!" Then, within a day or two, he slipped back into semi coma and died. His primary malignancy stemmed from smooth muscle cells gone wild in a section of smooth muscle in his bronchial tube, similar to the "smooth muscle tubes" for passage of bile. The patient had no history whatever of ever taking anabolic steroids, but had taken catabolic, anti-inflammatory steroids for asthma. What caused his condition and who can explain such peculiarities during management?

Charlie Roberts (Butt), UC Berkeley shot putter and discus thrower, was treated successfully for Hodgkin's Disease at Stanford medical center in Palo Alto California in 1975. His immune system, however, had to have been compromised from the treatments. Too soon after he died, at the early age of 40, from yeast pneumonia. There was no history of anabolic steroids. Had Charlie, my one time best friend in sports, used steroids, blame for his contracting Hodgkin's disease would have been placed on those anabolic hormones, not just by lay people but physicians as well.

Chicago Bears football sensation Walter Peyton died in his forties from a rare bile duct malignancy. Nobody knows why. Female track sensation, Flo Griffith Joyner reportedly died from sudden cardiac death, as have thousands of people. Had she been on thyroid medication, it would have been suspected as (somehow) causative, wouldn't it? There was no evidence of hypertrophic interstitial sub-aortic stenosis brought to my attention. Sudden cardiac deaths have occurred countrywide not too infrequently. Another lady suffered a sudden cardiac death, after she unexpectedly exacerbated into a manic psychosis. No steroids were involved, and anyway, it's difficult to even imagine steroids have much to do with cardiac conduction properly influencing the ventricles. Of further interest, pertaining to our bizarre world of contemporary drug abuses, "sudden sniffing deaths" have been reported in conjunction with inhalants creating an urge to run, but wouldn't it be dimwitted to presume competitive sprinters inhale aromatic solvents to give them "an edge, via an 'urge' to run?"

Anabolic steroid side effects include fluid retention and acne. A detectable personality change or mood swing may be corrected with a diuretic! The "steroid rage," is due to fluid retention. (for pre menstrual "rages," have the wife or girl friend take a diuretic.) Virilization in women may occur that affects the fetus during pregnancy. Increase of body hair, clitoral size and libido can become a side effect. If deepening of the voice does occur, in females using anabolic steroids, it seems to remain even upon discontinuance of the medication. Anabolic steroids are useful prescriptions for girls growing undesirably too tall, since this speeds long bone (epiphyseal) closure, to try to terminate a further increase in height growth pattern. Testicular shrinkage and gynecomastia may occur in men. Tamoxiphen (Nolvadex) is a treatment for gynecomastia and, by the way, this medicine to block estrogen receptors, was used by male field athletes long before most people in the US were aware of being useful for treatment of certain breast cancers.

It's important that serious side effects caused by other drugs not be confused with anabolic steroids. In the nineteen seventies at a weight lifting meet near San Jose California, I stood right next to this extremely powerful weight lifter, while he appeared to be listening and talking to one of the pillars in the auditorium! A minute or two later he went on to press 450 pounds on the tournament platform! His behavior was very eccentric. From observation it seemed consistent with "amphetamine induced schizophrenia," as alluded earlier. Various street drugs have provoked delusions as well as hallucinations. Cortisone type steroids, not anabolic but catabolic (break down tissue), anti-inflammatory and "suppressing" the immune system have uncommonly induced delusions and hallucinations: an "organic" psychosis. These "immune system suppressing" steroids have proven life saving in a variety of acute disease situations!

No sooner was I convinced "premature aging was the price paid for anabolic steroid usage," into my office came a well known physique star for some discussion about his steroid program and comment on his elevated serum cholesterol level and blood pressure. He reportedly used anabolic steroids for many years, yet he looked considerably younger than his stated age! He had experimented, learned to use Anavar for developing strength, Deca- Durabolin injections to get rid of subcutaneous fat, increasing "definition or cuts," and relied upon Testosterone injections for increasing muscular size.

His program at the time consisted of 20 hours per week devoted to training. He was taking Parabolin by mouth each day with injections biweekly of 1cc Testosterone and 1cc Deca-Durabolin for ten consecutive weeks followed by a drug holiday of six weeks. Both his serum cholesterol and his blood pressure were higher than hospital committee meetings and television ads allowed but certainly within an "expected range for athletes on anabolic steroid regimes." What he needed was reassurance. There was a good deal more to arterial blockage than elevated serum cholesterol. It was emphasized "cholesterol" was a substrate with acetic acid for adrenal cortex cells to synthesize all salt retaining, anti inflammatory, and anabolic hormones in those tissues. He was reassured "cholesterol" was essential for integrity of the membranes of all nucleated body cells, as well as for the production of bile for digestion. Since he was taking his anabolic hormones by mouth and injection, receptors on cells that produce anabolic hormones no doubt were less sensitive to bringing cholesterol from the circulation into the interior of those cells not inclined to make more still than he needed. Consistent heavy weight training has been shown for decades to reasonably elevate arterial blood pressure and often, with huge arms, a special cuff has been necessary for obtaining a correct measurement anyway. Blood pressure readings that became a neurosis by the late nineteen sixties have mislead many a patient starting them on the path of taking some medication they never needed. Commercialism!

As soon as it was evident anabolic steroid usage permitted the competitor to train virtually "full time," sports logically should have been divided into two separate bodies:

   1. Amateur Sports for enjoyment only

   2. Full Time Occupation Sports (Competitors on
     Anabolic steroid hormone programs.)

What was the sense of adopting a "Ban" on medications that enable the ambitious world class athlete to change from amateur status to full time jock? If an athlete's desire was to make his or her career full time and he or she was good enough at performing an athletic event to earn a living, why make this chosen "occupation," whether you like it or not, illegal? Ignoring facts has never made a fact go away! The public has already come to expect sensational (!) marks, records in sports only made possible with full time training which necessitates anabolic steroids! Where has their arisen "a desire to place a ban on higher, faster and heavier?" The military hasn't done it! NASA hasn't done it! Why has there been since 1974 this relentless targeting of the athletes?

It's completely agreed taking anabolic steroids, growth hormone, or anything else that works is unnecessary if you engage in athletics as an amateur! If however you have devoted yourself to individual competition that requires great muscular exertion and you "qualify," and wish to become world class what other option have you? You cannot work out full time, like a job, without exogenous anabolic assistance, because your muscular system can't handle it. You'll get "stale, depressed, and just collapse if you engage in continuous daily heavy barbell, dumbbell or weight throwing activity without such medication. Weight training has become an adjunct for football, boxing, baseball, and tennis. It all began with Track and Field in the U.S. in 1953. Anabolic programs have not helped reaction times or coordination, like Ping-Pong where you need blinding speed to return the ball. You had best wear goggles if you take on the Chinese!

While the Anabolic Steroid Ban of 1974 fell short of causing "a re-run of prohibition," it nevertheless made use of anabolic hormones "illegal," and changed what had been going on into a world wide crime wave! Behind the scenes preferential treatment kept the 1976 Montreal Olympic Games intact. The cost of those Games threatened the city of Montreal with bankruptcy, payments being made to this day! As soon as those 1976 Games ended, it was International Police, Border Guards and the FBI all involved in a chase for that little blue pill I once prescribed during internship for elderly fractured bone cases in 1958! By 1977 God must have wished he had allowed some of the human species better ability to reason. In spite of the terribly unjust testing of just one of every six athletes, not randomly but "politically," to show the "Ban" was "respected," the 1976 Games, a few athletes out of luck, proved a wonderful example of East versus West competition. After so very many years of intense training, Bruce Jenner edged the powerful Russian barely winning the decathlon exemplified by that cover shot on Sports Illustrated. Had the United States athletes been allowed to compete in Moscow in 1980 those Olympic Games would have been better yet! Brezhnev in the stands with a flask of vodka; he would have been delighted with the prospect of fair East-West competition, especially US v. Russia, and Henry Kissinger by rights should have been sitting right there next to him. (So much for pipe dreams.)

Whether you exercise your brain or your muscles there are no short cuts and you must either "pump your neurons or those skeletal muscles." Anabolic hormones and presumably growth hormone promote quicker skeletal muscle recovery. There is more rapid synthesis of new muscle in response to the increased amount of muscular work employed, during all those hours devoted each week to serious training.

For endurance competition the word's out about a sialic acid containing protein in the body called erythropoietin. This is natures' stimulator of production of immature, nucleated, red blood cells, the precursors that make more mature red blood cells available for oxygen carrying power. The mature red blood cells are without a nucleus and live 120 days. In the good old days simply training at high altitude serves the goal of increased oxygen carrying capacity since more red bloods cells are produced in response to the higher altitude. If the big competition is scheduled at sea level where there's 97% oxygen saturation, you temporarily have more red blood cells to work for you at that level of increased oxygen carrying power.

About 1 percent of oxygen saturation is lost per 1000 feet of altitude, so at 5000 feet you experience 92% oxygen saturation. At any rate epoetin alfa Epogen, a 165 amino acid glycoprotein produced naturally in one's kidney, (thus "ortho-molecular" coining a term of Linus Pauling), is very well tolerated by cyclists. Cyclists, of course, are anything but anemic! It's "illegal," to engage in "doping," and all I know from hearsay is that it is well tolerated, and it works! I am unable to advise cyclists and depend upon them to teach me about all this. The sport is so grueling it makes cardiologists more respectful for what the heart muscle can do! Upon learning from cyclists a physician can reason things out much better than a lawyer, judge or a petite jury. Listen to the patient I was taught, then form a judgment.

The power packs of cells, or mitochondria that utilize glucose and oxygen to release carbon dioxide and water respond to increased time and effort in sports training. Watch what you do if you are out of shape! You can become acutely overheated, brain cells are damaged at 107 degrees, and body temperature is "expectedly 104 in a well-trained athlete after running a mile." Working out constantly more than you should you become "stale" and lose the urge to train. Anabolic steroid hormones, oral or injected, "only make it possible to train longer." You may bounce back for more after as much as five hours per day six days per week (!), 52 weeks of the year if that is what you want to do! If you take anabolic steroids and then go to a movie, by not "using up" your prescription you may get into trouble and worse yet there's no benefit!

Any prescription drug can be acutely or chronically dangerous. Careless prescribing is one of the main concerns confronting the medical profession especially nowadays. Compared to certain drugs commonly prescribed anabolic hormones have a very wide margin of safety, evidenced by so many athletes who have consumed much more than necessary. Digitalis, a familiar prescription drug to strengthen the heart, has a very narrow margin of safety. In other words the adjusted dosage that is ideally effective is very close to the dosage that causes toxic very serious side effects. How many canines have gone to premature graves as a result of veterinarians using digitalis preparations?

The unfortunate belief anabolic steroid hormones have been classified as dangerous, if not soon then later, stems in part from a Chicago osteopathic college researcher. He recorded the testimony of a sports medicine specialist of Olney Maryland exclaiming such users of these anabolic hormones down the line will pay a terrible price! This interview made news in the Los Angeles Times on Wednesday, February 1, 1984.

The term "roid rage" became popular by 1987. This catchy description of explosive moods associated with anabolic steroids began with a Harvard professor of psychiatry who treated just two male anabolic hormone users. Both had "psychiatric problems!" Changing levels of both female hormones, estrogen and progesterone have been documented in relationship to fluid retention ("wet brain") relieved by a diuretic and uterine cramping relieved by judicious use of ibuprofen (Motrin). Why hasn't "the wrong time of the month been called "roid rage?" Millions of women have taken birth control pills to prevent pregnancy. Forgetting pregnancy, taking extra amounts of these very pills has made it possible for women to train harder and longer "legally!"

Sprint sensation Ben Johnson was singled out and humiliated world wide for anabolic steroid usage at the Olympic Games of 1988 in Seoul, South Korea. He ran the 100meter dash the fastest of anyone up to that time. People watching the Seoul Games were persuaded all other competitors were innocent! One official came across on television as if he had identified the one competitor of the 1988 Games that used anabolic hormones! Indirectly implied was that no other sprinter had trained with anabolic steroids but Ben Johnson!

At the Olympic Games 2000 held in Sydney Australia officials went further yet. They made sure the press got information to embarrass the recognized world shot put champion who had not recovered from injury enough to even compete in the 2000 Olympics! Of all things newspaper releases, supposedly focused on the Games, instead engaged every ones attention by featuring CJ Hunter testing positive for Nandrolone in Oslo Norway earlier in the summer of 2000. No one dared report the furthest the 16 pound shot was ever thrown by anyone without training with anabolic steroids was 60 feet ten inches. No reporter wrote, "Anabolic steroids, birth control pills, were used by female athletes" who were competing in the Sydney Games. There was no urge to come clean and admit the last Olympic Games, anabolic steroid free, was London in 1948. What was supposed to be accomplished by all this? What was the intent of the press anyway? Was it to convince the public that the Australians ran a strict and steroid free Olympics? If they did what do you suppose the record book would show?

To appease the audience, and still uphold an ideal of a completely drug free Olympics, Francois Carrard director general of the International Olympic Committee supervising the 2000 Sydney Games conceded Andreea Raducan, Romanian gold medal winner, gained no competitive edge by taking a cold remedy to clear her nasal passages! Regardless, in order to satisfy those involved in what at times has become a fanatical enforcement of drug policy, Andreea was required to surrender her first place medal in the all-around gymnastics competition! Those enforcing the rules went further. The "physician," who prescribed the cold remedy to clear her nasal passages, was suspended for five years!

Whether world class sports promoters and sports politicians believe it they do convey an opinion to the public that athletes, by getting plenty of sleep, training hard and eating properly can heave a 16 pound steel ball over 70 feet, hurl a disc 225 feet or jerk 500 pounds overhead. Regardless most know this is not anywhere near the case and so athletes are forced to continue to develop ways of outsmarting urine test authorities.

Athletes, using Testosterone, pre-test themselves by taking also the correct amount of epi-Testosterone. The reason: a 6:1 (or lower) ratio of Testosterone, the effective anabolic hormone, to epi-Testosterone that has no measurable muscle building or recuperative effect, means the athlete passes and may compete. Another very well established means of beating detection of anabolic steroids in the urine involves taking probenecid, a nineteen fifties gout remedy. Probenecid "blocks" the renal tubular secretion of anabolic steroids just like it blocks penicillin secretion prolonging an increased level of the antibiotic. While a positive test for probenecid that does increase tubular secretion of uric acid may raise suspicion, an athlete is able to "legally claim" it's for prevention of an attack of gout. Well, that is the purpose of the drug, so what are you supposed to say?

Twenty years ago it was claimed there's no way to test athletes who might switch to injections of synthesized Growth Hormone in place of anabolic steroids. This was emphasized prior to the 1984 Los Angeles Olympic Games probably because anabolic steroid urine testers had gotten all that "clean Olympics publicity." If they tested everyone, and their tests were fool proof, the sponsors could envision the LA Games be remembered as the Olympians get together that permitted no records set of any kind except for urine testing! It was sad the Soviet team wasn't permitted to show up. In 1980 the US snubbed the Moscow Olympics, so the gesture was thought of as simply tit for tat.

It was of interest that Nichols Laboratories located 50 or so miles from Los Angeles in San Juan Capistrano California had been manufacturing comparatively inexpensive multiple test kits for a 70 amino acid peptide, somatomedin-C, shipping them as far away as Italy by '84 Olympic Games time. Somatomedin-C, known to be dependent on somatotropin (Growth Hormone), simply testing positive for a high level of biological activity of somadomedin provided excellent indirect evidence of Growth hormone being taken! So there "was" a test for growth hormone! Why was this relatively inexpensive method of testing overlooked?

People have wondered why track and field, from the beginning of major Olympics interest, didn't split off and form its own Games. Actually they did, or at least tried, and did so honestly and above board. In 1973 the first international professional track and field organization was formed under the name: "International Track Association." Their field star was Brian Oldfield who demonstrated a spectacular discus hurling technique to put the 16pound shot 75 feet! It boggled the mind how he managed such a toss. Brian Oldfield was featured on the cover of Sports Illustrated. Anabolic steroids were legal in 1973! Nobody complained of feeling ill from using these anabolic prescriptions to train professionally and set records crowds expected from professional track and field athletes.

Track and field had been a feature of the Olympic Games since their modern revival in 1896. In fact, a variation of track and field competition using war equipment was featured in the original Greek Olympics of 776 BC! This combined with so much terrible publicity associated with anabolic steroids spelled a short survival (financially) for professional track and field's independence. Urine testing provided such "negative hype!" "Healthy 'drug free' games" were hypocritically advertised as symbolic of "Olympic Games," absolutely true from 1896 to 1948 but not beyond. The idea of fostering drug free competition enhanced the imagination of track and field audiences led to believe "Wheaties" the breakfast cereal of champions was enough. Big wig sports promoters unable to run 200 meters to catch their airplane determined what was best in terms of selling admission tickets. Spectacular records already established were somehow going to be broken with enthusiasm for training on just regular good food and plenty of rest.

Approximately 100 drugs were to be screened for Olympic Games athletes! Manfred Donike of Germany and Arnold Beckett of England, were obsessed with a dream the Los Angeles 1984 Games were to be the "purest" ever. It was as if gold, silver and bronze were to be awarded to the group sponsoring the most sophisticated urine test. Dr. Anthony Daly of the US, as part of the international Olympic committee, insisted all athletes be tested for caffeine! This startling suggestion was at last over ruled but it took some doing. It didn't matter an art history professor from a Southern California campus drank 20 cups of coffee every day but could only put the shot five feet. Moreover it was disclosed from the testing that 40 cups of coffee or 80 cups of tea or chocolate was necessary for caffeine to show up on any test available as of 1984. "The testing for 100 drugs flap, that included strychnine," in high gear many months prior to the LA Games, got so threatening international Olympic committee president of the Los Angeles Games, Peter Ueberroth, must have considered how everything worked out so well as some kind of financial miracle.

When the US athletes were prevented from competing in the Moscow Games of 1980 and the Soviets in turn didn't show up for the Los Angeles Games of 1984, many had the impression the urine testers had frightened the Russians away. A war in Afghanistan had started, however, when guerrillas in Afghanistan began creating major trouble in 1978. That war lasted until Mikael Gorbachev pulled Soviet forces out in 1988. By 1984 the Afghanistan War had become a "nightmare for the Soviets," especially since the US was on the side of Afghanistan! This tragic situation, bewildering for Gorbachev, was more than enough for the Soviets to get their minds off Olympic Games. Were the Soviets supposed to be enthusiastic for sports competition in Los Angeles under such wartime conditions?   President Jimmy Carter's foreign policy showed by hindsight a lack of foresight. My grandmother, Laura Gillespie, 100 years old in l980, a farm woman that voted a straight democratic ticket since the early nineteen twenties, was so upset with President Carter's policies, she, not seeing very well but hearing Ronald Reagan on television exclaimed, "I kind of like that Reagan!" I just happened to be talking with her on the telephone at the time. Her youngest son, Garnett Gillespie, laughed so hard at her comment he nearly fell limp to the floor. (I didn't make this up.)

In America, however, it was drugs and drug testing that received major publicity. Periodicals in magazines such as Good Housekeeping, Psychology Today and American Health labeled anabolic steroid hormones, "Rambo drugs." Women's breasts were shrinking! Men's sperm counts were dropping! "Rages," associated with anabolic steroids, had taken the place of Twinkys as a form of legal defense.

Spectators were not going to be pleased with records dropping as much as 20%! Athletes, engaged in sports for a living, were not about to accept any suggestion of returning to the days when Avery Brundage emphasized strictly "amateur' athletic competition. NASA gave no indication of giving up whatever proved necessary to safely send perfectly willing "space men and women" to Mars!

The 2004 Olympic Games is going to be about competition for breaking records, not lifting or tossing "less" or running and swimming "slower!" Training programs must enable these great athletes to perform in a manner to meet audience expectations. For that manned round trip to Mars, involving a year in space, something more for space persons than anabolic steroids is going to absolutely necessary. There's no question about it. For conditions on Earth where professional sports competition takes place, while that spaceship travels outwards, why continue with some Ban for athletes? There is no ban for necessary medications for space personnel? To help rid the Ban why can't athletes who took anabolic steroids or Growth Hormones confess; show the evidence no harm occurred? Certainly there's plenty of examples.

There was some very illegal activity associated with obtaining needed anabolic steroids if you believe some of the stories. World caliber athletes around San Jose California in the early nineteen seventies were pretty much in charge of their own prescriptions. Was a container ship with vast stores of Halotestin and other such drugs really hijacked in the South China Sea? Did a freight car sized container accidentally go overboard to be picked up as a planned action? At any rate that amount of anabolic steroids including Squibb's Halotestin brand of fluoxymesterone reportedly wound up in that area of California. Those products became available to athletes quite reasonably obviating any need for some nervous doctor to write a prescription.

Why did even endocrinologists desert the athletes? Why was political correctness allowed to scare interested physicians away from prescribing what world class athletes determined necessary? It was either get what you need or quit high level competitive sports which meant looking for another line of work. In retrospect the "Ban" was a sociological mistake. Making anabolic hormone prescriptions illegal for athletes was based on armchair opinions and judgments lacking first hand experience. Why did certain physicians collaborate then lead the way making something illegal that, if stopped, spelled the end of world class sports as we over the years have come to know it? What was the sense for making legal drugs suddenly "illegal?"

As they say natures abhors a vacuum. By the nineteen eighties the void, left by physicians frightened from helping athletes, was filled by a Los Angeles college theatrical major and a popular body builder by the name of Dan Duchaine. Based on his clinical experience that out shined any physician's, with so many involved with taking anabolic steroids, he determined they were reasonably safe to recommend. Dan Duchaine put out a guidebook that was well received, very much appreciated and improved upon as time and experience went on.

One physician and former athlete was sympathetic to the needs of the super jocks. His name was Robert Kerr. He tried to fill the void and manage athletes on anabolic steroids but there were so many! What he did was follow each one with liver enzyme tests using such findings as an early warning signal for significant side effects. Dr. Kerr was also sought after by television producers to air his viewpoint. The international Olympic committee members reacted by accusing Kerr of simply enjoying the limelight. Some athletes complained (to me) Dr. Kerr was unable to spend any time to answer their questions but, 24 hours in each day, how could he?

The hype over dangers associated with anabolic steroids was thought of as an over reaction lacking common sense. Athletes learned as they felt their way along. They also learned overworking their skeletal muscles with anabolic steroids led in some cases to myoglobinuria. When their kidneys were unable to get rid of "excess oxygen transporting storage protein called myoglobin" dialysis, understandably though uncommonly, proved necessary. A great number of athletes took anabolic steroid recipes for many years without any difficulty.

It's over 50 years since the Russians began administering Testosterone shots or placing Testosterone pellets under the skin to find out if this enabled top athletes to train harder and longer. There are those within the international Olympic committee that have remained skeptical about anabolic steroid usage making any difference. It's a wonderment why some resist understanding it's the ability to train harder and longer that put so many records where they are.

NASA has learned anabolic steroids work like the Russians showed us. NASA has also learned something more than those anabolic steroids will prove necessary for space travelers, to keep anti gravity muscles in shape, during prolonged periods of weightlessness or zero gravity. For those who have agreed to accept the risk of a round trip to Mars is it to be expected they will be called "cheats" and "fools" for needing certain medications to hopefully make their trip a success?

No one referred to cosmonaut Valery Polyakov, or astronaut (US Senator) John Glenn as a cheat or fool. When someone has accomplished something you would not dare to try, interpersonal relationships within society improve by showing some appreciation. Behind such great efforts has always been reasonable purpose.

In Rome Italy during the 1988 Seoul Korea Olympic Games, newspapers featured many sports articles about the Games. One newspaper used terms like, "potenza esplosiva," and "rapida combustione!" Italians have had reason to laugh at American dietary fads that seem to them extreme one way or another. They have room to laugh. Italians have three years life expectancy over the US due to cooking with olive oil, sedating their disruptive toddlers with a swig of wine, eating a lot of pizza, handling stress better, or who knows? Regarding the Olympic Games held in Seoul, Italians were especially curious how certain American female athletes had become so powerful! In the sports section of Il Messaggero, September 16, page 19, a report attempted to satisfy this question, "How was it possible Florence Griffith Joyner ran 100 meters in 10.4 seconds? Past records were recorded in the article for reference:

1927:	Gertrud Gladitsch, (Germany),	100 meter dash:	12.1 seconds
1988:	Flo Griffith Joyner (USA),	100 meter dash:	10.4 seconds

Difference: 1.7 seconds!

1927:	Charlie Paddock (USA),	100 meter dash:	10.2 seconds
1988:	Ben Johnson (Canada),	100 meter dash:	9.83 seconds

Difference: only 0.37 seconds!

There were no anabolic steroids in 1927 when Charlie Paddock ran his spectacular 100meter dash! Charlie Paddock has remained, in the minds of some elderly sports fans, as the greatest natural sprinter. Roger Bannister has continued to be thought of as the greatest miler. Babe Ruth has remained the best baseball player by many serious fans of baseball. None of these champions took anabolic steroids! There were none to take! They trained seriously but comparatively speaking utilized only a fourth or a third as much invested time as the champions of today.

During the newspaper coverage of the 1988 Olympics it was disclosed Ben Johnson tested positive for anabolic steroid hormones. This for the Italians accounted for his running the distance 0.37 seconds faster than Charlie Paddock. It was "understandable."

It was female athletic accomplishments that seriously engaged the interest of Italians. Over a span of 61 years, how was it "girls managed to improve, relatively speaking, four to five times more than the guys?" That was the question! The logical answer was that female athletes have been training longer and harder on anabolic steroid hormone assisted training programs as well!

As of 1956 oral medications known as birth control pills have been available consisting usually of two anabolic steroids. While recommended daily dosages, as prescribed, prevented pregnancy, larger dosages made it possible to train longer and harder and modifications of those molecular structures have been used by female athletes.

Has the medical profession distanced itself from the truth of the matter? In the middle nineteen eighties Allan J. Ryan, editor of "Physician and Sports Medicine," had put in print what I felt was a baffling statement: "Anabolic Steroids are ineffective and do not work at all." His publication went on to say: "Those who thought anabolic hormones were effective have not read

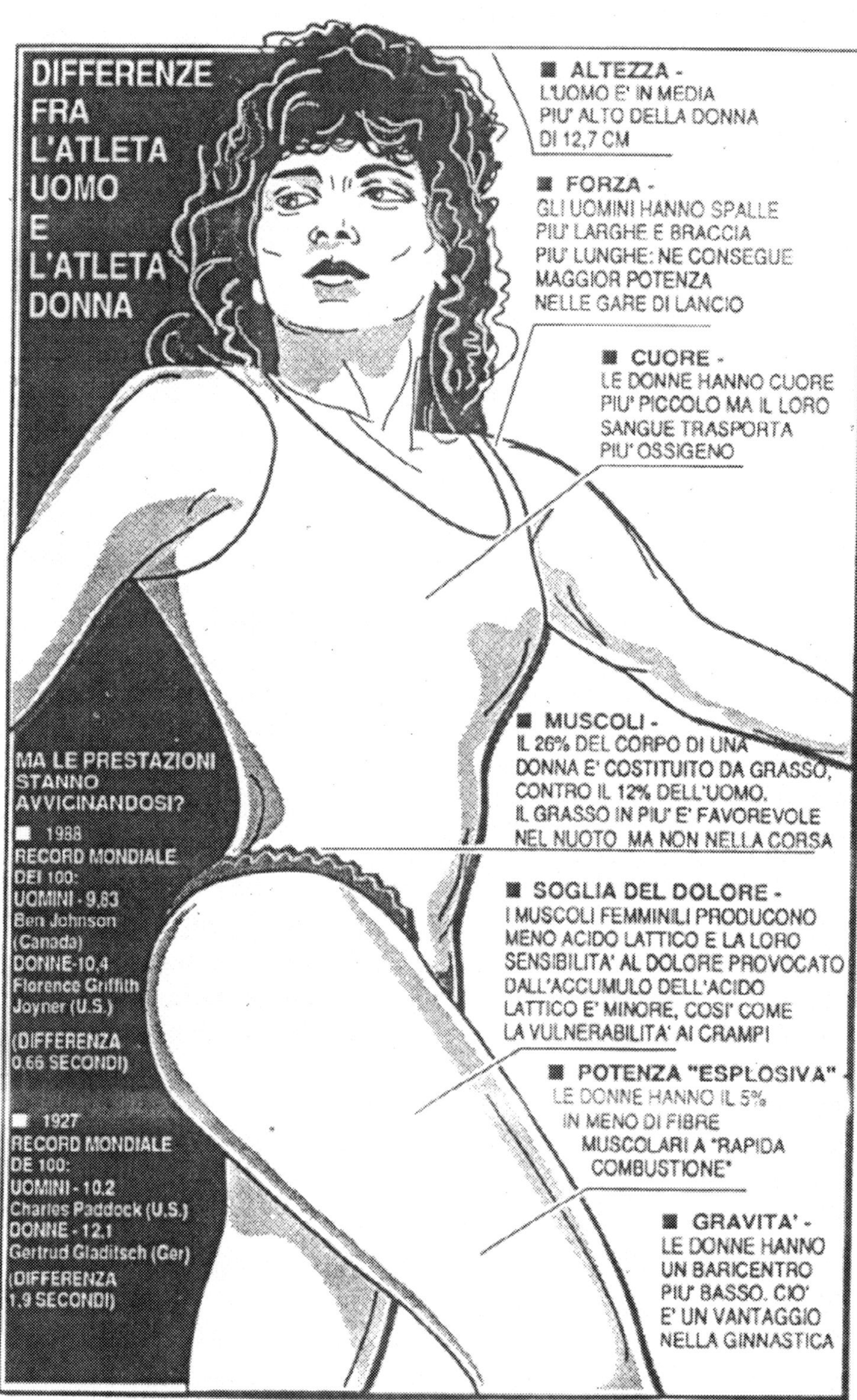
IL MESSAGGERO
VENERDI'
16 SETTEMBRE 1988
19

DIFFERENZE
FRA
L'ATLETA
UOMO
E
L'ATLETA
DONNA

MA LE PRESTAZIONI
STANNO
AVVICINANDOSI?
1988
RECORD MONDIALE
DEI 100:
UOMINI - 9,83
Ben Johnson
(Canada)
DONNE -10,4
Florence Griffith
Joyner (U.S.)

(DIFFERENZA
0,66 SECONDI)

1927
RECORD MONDIALE
DE 100:
UOMINI - 10.2
Charles Paddock (U.S.)
DONNE - 12.1
Gertrud Gladitsch (Ger)
(DIFFERENZA
1,9 SECONDI)

ALTEZZA -
L'UOMO E' IN MEDIA
PIU' ALTO DELLA DONNA
DI 12,7 CM

FORZA -
GLI UOMINI HANNO SPALLE
PIU' LARGHE E BRACCIA
PIU' LUNGHE: NE CONSEGUE
MAGGIOR POTENZA
NELLE GARE DI LANCIO

CUORE -
LE DONNE HANNO CUORE
PIU' PICCOLO MA IL LORO
SANGUE TRASPORTA
PIU' OSSIGENO

MUSCOLI -
IL 26% DEL CORPO DI UNA
DONNA E' COSTITUITO DA GRASSO,
CONTRO IL 12% DELL'UOMO.
IL GRASSO IN PIU' E' FAVOREVOLE
NEL NUOTO MA NON NELLA CORSA

SOGLIA DEL DOLORE -
I MUSCOLI FEMMINILI PRODUCONO
MENO ACIDO LATTICO E LA LORO
SENSIBILITA' AL DOLORE PROVOCATO
DALL'ACCUMULO DELL'ACIDO
LATTICO E' MINORE, COSI' COME
LA VULNERABILITA' AI CRAMPI

POTENZA "ESPLOSIVA"
LE DONNE HANNO IL 5%
IN MENO DI FIBRE
MUSCOLARI A "RAPIDA
COMBUSTIONE"

GRAVITA' -
LE DONNE HANNO
UN BARICENTRO
PIU' BASSO. CIO'
E' UN VANTAGGIO
NELLA GINNASTICA

Folla
scatenata
per
l'arrivo
di Steffi

Migliaia
di tifosi
coreani
hanno accolto
con calore
persino
eccessivo
la tennista
tedesca
Steffi Graf
all'aeroporto,
ignorando
altri campioni.
Steffi
s'è spaventata

t

The 'research' carefully." Presumably Allan Ryan had not considered the purpose of the anabolic hormones. The sole purpose was to triple heavy weight training time. Obviously if one fails to put in that extra time taking the medicines would not make any significant difference. When those comments were actually published it raised wonderment how many physicians worldwide, who have read or read one or some of the 3000 medical journals published in the world, have been exposed to opinions that have failed by a long shot to reflect their own personal experience(s). Such wonderment has remained as of 2003 especially after more than a decade of so much commercialization.

What is the truth? What is "truth" by the way? The truth is there are times when it may be best not to just blurt out the truth. One needs wisdom. The use of wisdom truthfully improves the stabilization of interpersonal relationships that make up society. Temperance is very important to keep things calm. When any physician faces a patient with what's believed to be a fatal illness and the patient says, "Give it to me straight!" Some physicians reportedly do that, however, from my training that is not the proper thing to do. Instead you cautiously provide some ray of hope and reveal your frank opinion to that person closest to the patient. The truth, provided what you have been persuaded to believe actually becomes the truth, may be revealed later on, or, at a more strategically ideal time.

The captain of a passenger liner is notified his ship's hull is damaged, leaking badly, and the bilge systems cannot keep up. The ship is due to sink within four hours! A wise captain is not going to get on the speaker and say, "Now hear this, I'm just informed this ship is going to sink in four hours!" That may be the truth however, using wisdom and temperance, maybe he'll announce "a surprise life jacket drill as a recent requirement for cruise lines," one "unannounced life boat drill is currently required sometime while at sea." In this way panic is minimized and so will injuries and loss of life. (That's the truth!)

Before cosmonauts and astronauts are launched to Mars, the truth about matters on Earth that concern top level worldwide competitive sports should be revealed. Knowledgeable physicians, lawyers, Olympic committee members, sports promoters and especially world class athletes of past and present should come forward. If those involved in urine testing succeed in making urine testing the major behind the scenes Olympic event then let 'em! But let's oppose this and hope for a smooth transition, once and for all, from those times gone forever remembered as the "Age of Breakfast Cereals and Amateur Sports" to the present. Let's philosophically adjust to the present where excelling in sports not only means a college scholarship but also a full time job! "The Age of Anabolic Steroids makes possible the Age of the Full Time Athlete." For those at the top it becomes an occupation. It's already that way. Why not accept it?

Oh, by the way, when you mention steroids it is very important to be very specific. Vitamin D is a "steroid!" Vitamin D is a "hormone" that was mistakenly classified as a "vitamin" many decades ago. Too much of it, by the way "can kill you," although that means hundreds of thousands to millions of units, the latter for instance contained as is Vitamin A in polar bear liver, not likely a part of any ones diet, certainly not one among the fads of athletes.

Speculating about disease prevention perhaps anyone, who as a child received a daily spoon full of cod liver oil, unwittingly benefits by that source of nutrition that conceivably helps prevent heart disease and, some believe, certain forms of cancer later on. As of 2003 some investigators believe hormone D is vital in regards to cell division and cell death. Some say adequate amounts of Vitamin D help prevent cancer of the breast, prostate, ovary and colon. Is there really any 'truth' to this? The truth is nobody really knows, but it has engaged some attention.

Where hormone D and the skin are concerned it's rightly considered very important to avoid sunburn! Sunlight (ultra violet B rays), via minutes exposure for fair skinned, in contrast to hours for dark skinned persons, converts cholesterol in skin to an inactive hormone, vitamin D that then needs two hydroxyl (OH) groups, gathered in the liver and kidneys, to become: 1,25 hydroxy Vitamin ("steroid hormone") D! This steroid hormone D, however, may also easily be obtained from dietary sources, especially cereals, fortified milk and fleshy fatty fish like salmon. There's always "fish liver oil," however my childhood memories just won't allow it! Ugh!

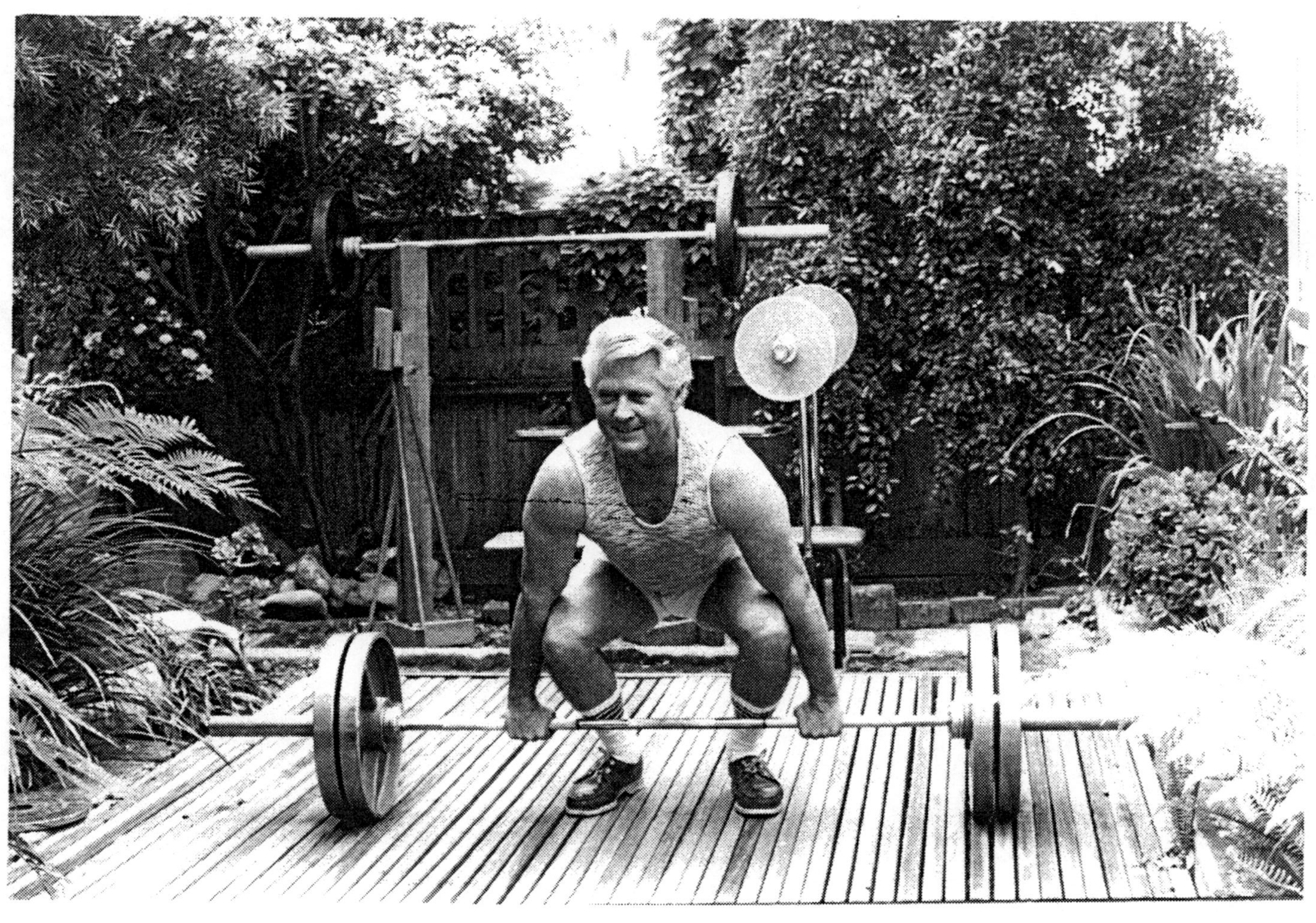

AUTHOR HOISTING THE "IRON PILLS" ON LAGUNA BEACH
PROPERTY   17th YEAR SOLO PRACTICE
Never Took Steroids

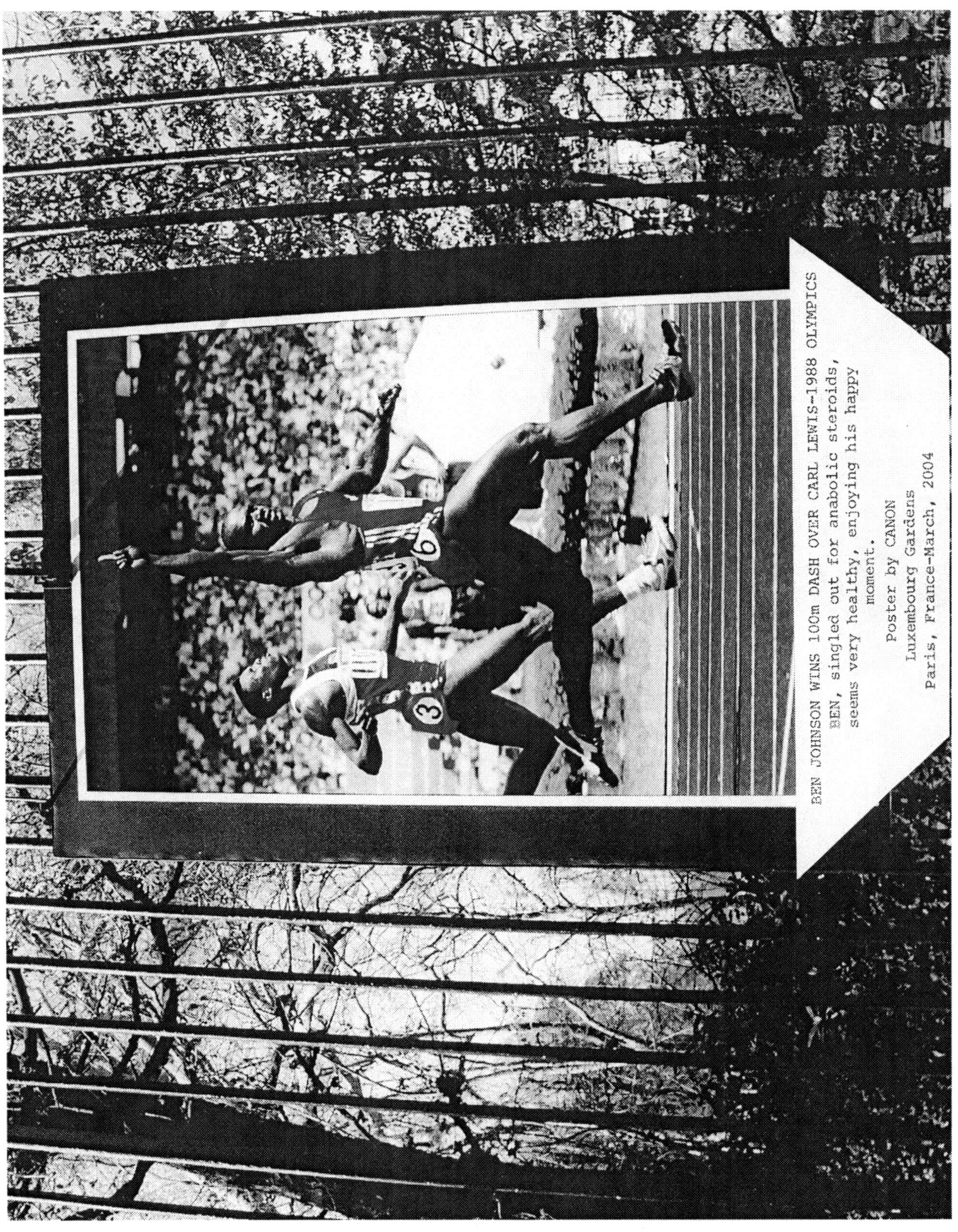

BEN JOHNSON WINS 100m DASH OVER CARL LEWIS~1988 OLYMPICS
BEN, singled out for anabolic steroids,
seems very healthy, enjoying his happy
moment.

Poster by CANON
Luxembourg Gardens
Paris, France~March, 2004

CHAPTER V

PSYCHIATRISTS CHALLENGE MENTAL ILLNESS

How to recognize and handle "abnormal people" has been a problem since mankind began. From what is extant and by using ones' imagination the history of this challenge has been reconstructed and documented by persons, of course, who were not there. Through logic it's been inferred, the very moment communication took place, there was fear and suspicion. Peace of mind proved relaxing. Any unusual disturbance, robbing one of a peaceful feeling, was probably considered evil. Interpersonal relationships, leading to feelings of comfort and relaxation, and increased confidence, were good. Certain individuals seemed more caring, and unselfish. They, accordingly, transferred confidence to others. Due to ignorance and superstition witches, in considerable numbers, were burned at the stake. Sorcerers were hung. Much has been carefully documented about sorcery, witchcraft and superstition.

On the Isle of Capri in 1987, with friend and retired professor of Latin languages, Stanley Bonner of England, (books include, "The Origin of Oratory in the Roman Empire," University. of California press), Stanley pointed out a cliff above us as we came ashore by boat. Emperor Tiberius, he explained, lived sometimes at the top in his villa. Tiberius, stepson of the first Rome emperor, became the second emperor of Rome when Caesar Augustus (Octavian) died in A.D.14. (Octavian was the nephew of Julius Caesar, master of Rome, who died in 44B.C.). Tiberius, for "amusement," Stanley said, had various persons perform "running long jumps off the cliff," starting their run on the villa grounds, with the finish line 800 feet below! The unlucky person, most probably a Christian who refused to grant divine honors to the emperor, was told to get up as much speed as possible, because, otherwise, he would be snagged at the edge to be penalized via a much harsher death! Emperor Tiberius, based on what I learned, was kinder than Emperor Caligula (A.D.37–A.D. 41), and much kinder than the stepson of Claudius (who was busy being dominated by his wives), called Nero! (A.D.54-A.D.68). Christians, felt as an ever increasing "problem for Rome," Nero simply ordered a barbarous execution of many of them, including St. Peter and St. Paul. Was "mental illness" involved in all this? Or was it just a matter of insisting on "freedom" on the one hand, and a case of maintaining "law and order," on the other, with nobody on either side able to demonstrate a better way to go about peacefully solving their problem?

Early on people sampled what we call herbs from non-woody plants. From leaves and buds, even from bark of some trees, from tasting, nibbling or sampling, either you poisoned yourself, got sick, perhaps died, or, you stumbled on to something you could chew or swallow that tasted good or, in some way, made you feel better, perhaps really got you going!

Just imagine having returned to your dwelling, to discover your family and neighbors had sampled something that made them act in a very strange manner. As you reached out to embrace your mate she gnashes her teeth and bites off the end of your finger! Unfortunately she had eaten some of the seed of rye grass containing too much of a fungus now known as ergot. Others were drinking their own urine, which perhaps wasn't that unusual! The substance that caused that type of organic psychoses among the group was, by today's knowledge, the alkaloid known as belladonna. On a more pleasant note that same alkaloid, obtained from a perennial herb, with dark purple flowers and shining purplish-black berries, dilated a lady's pupils making her more beautiful.

There was a need for a "medicine man" or "shaman," who may have been as ignorant of all the goings on as everyone else, his special value being he cared more about those persons suffering from unfortunate mistakes, or, unrecognizable diseases. By conveying such concern for those who recovered, he was given credit for having magical powers.

Beginning as a student, under the legendary French artist and neurologist, Jean Martin Charcot (1825-1893), Viennese professor of neuropathology, Sigmund Freud (1856-1939), took a special interest in abnormal behavior. He began observing forms of paralysis. He also studied and observed the loss of ability to name familiar people, or objects (aphasia), and, he attempted to establish a relationship between hysteria and epilepsy, particularly opisthotonos, with the body resting on head and heels, a result of strychnine poisoning. Freud explored hypnosis as a means of determining the "why" of various conditions. He looked into the content of dreams to explain the "why" of forms of insanity. Psychoanalysis began as Freud traced symptoms of hysteria to psychic trauma earlier in life. He speculated such resulted in previously unreleased emotional energy to cause "conversion" (hysteria). Much came into view of a sexual nature. His method of therapy eventually known as "catharsis" emphasized free association, and he eventually discovered that preferable to hypnosis.

The ability to recognize all kinds of abnormal behavior, as well as handle those with such trouble, was far from solved at the start of the 20th century. It was an institutionalized patient's autobiography titled, "A Mind That Found Itself," written by Clifford Beers that engaged great interest.   Adolph Meyers, neurologist and psychiatrist at Cornell and Johns Hopkins, was particularly struck by Beer's experience. A concept of "mental hygiene" was introduced, and by 1908 there was considerable public interest. With Adolph Meyers' encouragement a national committee for mental hygiene was formed in 1909, the same year acclaimed educator, Abraham Flexner, provided the American Medical Association with the "Flexner Report of 1909." This report became a milestone for instituting improvements in the methods medical students were taught to become doctors.

During the latter part of the 19th century anecdotes, gathered from the observation of colonized mentally ill patients, resulted in useful information. Julius Wagner von Jauregg documented cases of psychotic behavior that seemed improved after experiencing a very high fever usually associated with malaria. By the late 19th and early 20th century it was observed that schizophrenics, who coincidentally had convulsive seizures, (no relationship, however, between the two conditions whatsoever) did improve following a generalized convulsion. By 1922, just a year after Banting and Best discovered insulin, it was learned that too great a dosage of insulin resulted in a precipitous fall in blood glucose, sufficient to provoke a very severe generalized seizure. Manfred Sakel utilizing such observations developed "insulin (seizure) coma therapy," by 1927, in order to treat and improve the psychotic state of patients. And there were benefits!

By the mid nineteen thirties, based on the pioneering work of Portugese professor of neurology and political diplomat Egas Moniz (1874-1955), who in 1949 shared the Nobel prize in medicine and physiology with WR Hess, an approach to otherwise seemingly unconquerable mental illness known as "lobotomy" was developed. The most successful method involved a severing of just frontal lobe nerve fibers, connected in part to lower centers of the brain, particularly the thalamus and brain stem. While this procedure, between 1936 and 1956, was performed in skilled hands quite simply and rapidly, it disappointingly resulted in a vegetative state rather than merely a calming effect about 50% of the time, and thus was phased out in favor of the new drug breakthrough, Thorazine and electro-convulsive-therapy (ECT).

It was in 1938 Cerletti and Bini of Italy developed and introduced ECT. A brief pulsation sufficient to light a 20watt bulb for two seconds became standardized. By 1956 the introduction of succinylcholine, a drug given prior to ECT that very temporarily blocked skeletal muscle movements, made ECT a smoothly administered non traumatic treatment in skilled hands.

Psychiatrists experienced in ECT became aware of its immense benefit in properly selected cases. It quickly became the treatment of choice for "change of life (involutional) depression." The post ECT amnesia, that typically erased two to four weeks of memory prior to ECT therapy, often times proved to be of additional benefit and even a blessing, in conjunction with success eliminating depression, resulting from a series of ECT.

Unfortunately those involved with contemporary forms of drug abuse, who steadfastly denied it, and gave totally untruthful medical histories, (especially "spent shells" representing post amphetamine usage depression), were given ECT and made worse! By the nineteen seventies a sister of a California legislator hospitalized in a mental health facility at Atascadero represented one such case. As a result, state legislation was passed requiring three psychiatric opinions for "legal permission to administer ECT." In addition, a judge's approval was required after the three opinions were obtained! Those involved, passing the law, were unaware that expertly timed ECT, even a couple of treatments at the beginning, sometimes made a difference as dramatic as the necessary removal of an inflamed appendix! Yet, all too few practitioners were, for whatever reasons, supportive. The psychoanalytical arm of psychiatry failed to lend their support. Difficulties created by the new California state law, along with hippies, street drug users and abusers, along with Vietnam War protesters, all without enough knowledge to understand what they were doing, managed to discredit ECT. Once the bandwagon got rolling psychiatrists, and then even an Oregon neurologist got on board. This culminated in a protest march in front of the California capitol at Sacramento!

Personal experience with ECT from the late nineteen sixties through the seventies, confirms that at least 16 bilateral treatments, followed by two more spaced treatments to stabilize, are necessary for lasting benefits, with no need then for post ECT anti depressant medication!

My final personal experience with ECT was in the late nineteen seventies. A woman in her sixties, with a manifest severe manic mood disorder, paced for seven days and nights before two other psychiatric opinions and a judge's authorization were obtained. The patient could have experienced a sudden cardiac death as a result of these laborious requirements. 22 ECT treatments then cured her completely. She took a Mediterranean cruise with her daughter and experienced five more years of quality life.

By the nineteen eighties it seemed all psychiatrists became hesitant to employ ECT. Reportedly there were about 1500 legal actions taken against psychiatrists for administering ECT in the city of Chicago Illinois at any given time! Psychiatrists still tried to do what was best for their depressed patients. They continued to employ ECT, however, leery of malpractice actions, many patients were shortchanged. Afraid to stay with experiences of the past, "by giving a necessary 'full course' of shock treatments," those, that improved dramatically, were given only an average of eight treatments. Indeed most physicians were fearful of proceeding further for sake of being sued! The bad advice logically may have come from malpractice carriers threatened with bankruptcy. Some patients were given unilateral treatments that proved almost worthless. In Chicago, one lady I knew personally in her mid fifties dramatically improved on eight treatments. Through a telephone call, the sister of the ECT patient, became tearful, exclaiming she had never had such a normal conversation with her sister! Within weeks, not given sufficient treatments to clear the depression indefinitely, given an anti depressant and calming agent, doxepin, (Sinequan), the "shortchanged ECT patient" made her fourth suicide attempt successfully, and committed suicide with too much alcohol in combination with that medicine.

Up to 2003, no other therapy for depression has been more effective than ECT in properly selected cases. However, the psychiatrist must have the proper training and the confidence to know what he or she is doing. It's reported more than 80% of patients, who have benefited from ECT, have regarded their treatments, in retrospect, no more worrisome than a trip to their dentist! (It's true!)

How does ECT do the job? It's not known. Speculating, ECT works by altering ion fluxes. In the brain there's "an influx of certain ions and an efflux of others," such as in the heart. For that matter, no one understands the heart muscle completely, let alone the brain! We do know there are ions, fluxes, and "channels." Reduction (gathering electrons) and oxidation (giving up electrons to oxygen) is well established. Perhaps, in the future, psychiatrists will tell their depressed patients they are suffering from a "channelopathy," referring to some imbalance regarding sodium, calcium, potassium, or other brain transmitter ion channels. ECT can correct an imbalance. Perhaps a psychiatrist will advise a patient he or she has a problem with a "second messenger system," particularly one membrane bound protein called the G-protein. The G-protein is one of a few guanine nucleotide binding regulatory proteins, specifically "Gi," (inhibitory for adenyl cyclase), the most abundant G-protein in the brain. Even if such an explanation proves completely erroneous, at least the patient will be relieved, convinced their doctor is still studying!

Knowledge of depression, as we know it, comes first from the Eber papyrus of Egypt thousands of years ago. Also the Old Testament of the Bible refers to King Saul who is depressed. Fixing him up with a young woman proves unhelpful. Music helps a little. Finally Saul becomes enraged and attempts to kill both his son (David) and the musician! What Saul needs is ECT, but unfortunately such treatment is unavailable for another 2700 years! Both then and now it takes more to correct a case of depression than a pat on the back and the words, "cheer up!"

During 1949 and 1950 the National Institute, and the Association for Mental Health, respectively, were formed, as two bodies dedicated to mental illness research and overall care, along with public information pertaining to mental illness of all kinds.

With more and more mentally ill on the street, psychiatric social workers blame former governor of California, Ronald Reagan. For nearly 30 years, in California, the job exposure of the psychiatric workers has been anything but easy. Mentally ill have been free to roam and share time and experiences with chronic alcoholics and other drug abusers. This has led to one sad experience after another trying to deal with the homeless, the old, the too young, the sad and the lonely, to try and provide them with some food and safety on a daily basis. More unbearable, when a solution that eases every one's worries has been found, too often the person in need, at least in a way normal people see it, refuses to cooperate and, "legally," is not required to cooperate! What is the answer?

"Should California's giant mental hospitals be re opened, or should new such facilities be built?" First it needs to be known there was more to the sinful situation, escaping public scrutiny, that led to California's "Lanterman-Petris-Short Act," signed into law by Governor Ronald Reagan. It is true the law closed most of the state's huge institutions for the mentally ill, in part due to far too much "therapeutic optimism," (successes treating patients with the new drug, lithium). Mentally ill then become integrated into communities! Being personally acquainted with all three legislators, Frank Lanterman of La Canada, Nick Petris of Oakland, and Alan Short, of Stockton, and becoming friends with Frank Lanterman for a number of years, some of the outrageous goings on that needed fixing were related first hand. It is hopeful decisions to improve things overall were made. In some ways things are better, and in some ways things are worse. The answers for the mentally ill are just not coming along as one hoped.

Every conceivable kind of wrongdoing imaginable occurred within state mental hospitals! Not everyone who occupied the facilities had a mental disturbance. Elderly fathers and mothers were committed to these institutions that were not mentally ill! Daughters and sons, usually in cahoots with their spouses, together with cooperative attorneys "institutionalized a parent" to take control of the "uncooperative" parent's money!" Explosive arguments about financing, or keeping a business profitable, brought out misbehavior sufficient for court hearings, and resulted in judge's decisions, ruling the elderly parent was irrational and should be institutionalized! Bank accounts of the elderly were confiscated! Some such accounts were commingled between the institutionalized parent's offspring(s) and their lawyer. It was not unheard of for a judge's name to be placed on a confiscated bank account! Such goings on exemplified what Irish playwright George Bernard Shaw cleverly said, "lack of money is the root of all evil!"

Giant mental facilities closed or not George Bernard Shaw seems to be correct. County sheriffs continue to observe so called "on-going homicides" with the victim being an elderly parent, deprived of essential medication while living in the home of a married off spring. The sinister plot is typically to acquire, or gain control of, the parent's money! What exactly do elderly persons "do" to protect their assets; to maintain some ability when to decide to whom and how "to leave their assets behind?"

In the nineteen sixties, resulting from numerous personal conversations with Frank Lanterman, (R) La Canada, chairman of ways and means for the California legislature, this led to personal contact with Governor Ronald Reagan. It seemed evident to me Ronald Reagan, later as president of the US, wisely planned to seek federal funding to cope with so many mentally ill, particularly in California. With all their new freedoms there was an obvious need for more qualified personnel to address the "problems of mentally ill on the street." Nancy Reagan said, "Say no to drugs!" That was part of the problem.

Ironically in 1981 during his first year as president Reagan was shot in the chest at close range, by none other than a psychotic patient, and was barely saved before he bled to death! This event had a tremendous emotional impact upon Nancy Reagan. It also caused the United States Supreme Court to alter its view on how to better handle insane psychiatric patients who performed absolutely senseless acts. As for federal funding for the mentally ill, particularly in California, it continued to fall short. Somehow the focus on this problem that has worsened since the Reagan presidency has been lost.

As for more history on the medical treatment for the mentally ill, a wave of enthusiasm began as early as 1950. Rauwolfia Serpentina, or Reserpine, used in India for centuries, demonstrated a calming effect. (It also slowed the pulse and lowered blood pressure.) By 1952 this alkaloid was isolated and carefully studied. It sedated the patient but, of much greater interest, Reserpine to its detriment was found to deplete biologically active amines such as "serotonin," (from the dietary essenital amino acid, tryptophan) along with "dopamine," "nor adrenalin," and "adrenalin," all coming from tyrosine (derived from the dietary essential amino acid, phenyl alanine). This meant Reserpine was undesirable for long term usage by depleting essential biologically active amines.

One should not get the notion India or China leads the world in the application of useful remedies. In India, strychnine is still used as a stimulant, hardly a drug of choice. In India, sleeping pills are still employed to treat convulsive seizure symptoms, not a good idea, apt only to complicate the problem. Reportedly in China there have been observations about the effects of marijuana for over 5000 years (more concentrated forms are known as hashish and charas), otherwise known in the West as "weed, pot, dope, hemp, joint, reefer, root or roach." "Dope" best describes this ancient euphoriant, hallucinogen and sedative because, in perspective, only pharmacologically uneducated people believe it to be the most ideal treatment for anything. Trying to make it "selectively available," for some chronically ill to combat nausea and increase appetite is certainly reasonable but countrywide it is unrealistic to think this can be done without detrimental sociological effects.

There is medicinal value in marijuana. It is, for awhile, a dilator of pulmonary bronchial tubes as well as a calming agent, however, there is "tolerance" to consider. In other words more and more may be needed to maintain a desired effect. The reason the federal government is reluctant to legalize marijuana is because "widespread usage is destructive to 'society'." Is there a better reason than that? A so called "amotivational syndrome," or pervasive feeling of apathy, occurs with regular use of marijuana. Nothing seems to be important to the regular user! Is that beneficial to the very survival of the country?

Personally, I believe marijuana is a stepping stone to further drug abuse. It's typically first and most easily available for youngsters who desire to "party and modify their mental state." In addition, it is stored in fatty tissue, in the brain, causes brain wave activity to become abnormal. Since brains do not fully mature until about age 16, it doesn't make sense to take some product that doesn't belong in your brain while it is maturing. For the cardiovascular system marijuana is certainly not beneficial. It increases oxygen demands for the heart muscle while decreasing oxygen delivery (!), hardly something that anyone with athletic aspirations would want to be using. .

Bromide, introduced by Charles Locock in 1857, was quickly determined useful as a sedative and anti-convulsant in spite of its side effects including a rash, lethargy and mental confusion. It was Fischer and Von Mering in 1903 who discovered the spectacular breakthrough with the barbiturates, properly used for sedation and to combat seizure symptoms, being both effective and safe. Diazepam marketed under the familiar name, Valium, proved the ultimate calming agent for acute circumstances. It was introduced for use in practice in the US in l963. By 1977 the "diazepam receptor" was discovered in the brain which meant that the very substance created in the lab of Hoffman La Roche (Valium) proved to be identical to a product synthesized in the brain! This helped explain why patients were having difficulty getting off Valium since taking it regularly for too many weeks obviated need for the brain to synthesize it. It required a month or so to resume normal production in the brain, and thus a number of very anxious days of withdrawal trying to discontinue the drug.

In the nineteen seventies flurazepam (Dalmane), structurally related to Librium and Valium, marketed as a hypnotic to induce sleep proved more useful than any barbiturate for that purpose. Dalmane had low addiction potential and left intact rapid eye movement (REM) paradoxical sleep that represented about half of expectedly normal sleep. By not making demands on one's liver and with a so-called high therapeutic index making fatal poisoning unlikely Dalmane became recognized as a remarkably safe and effective drug, as true today as it was when introduced.

Who could predict Thalidamide, the most hypnotically potent sleeping pill ever released, with toxicity so low to make suicide nearly impossible, if taken, "just one dose between the 24th and 36th day of pregnancy," adversely would affect embryonic limb buds resulting in a deformed newborn with grotesque stubby limbs? (Phocomelia) The sociological impact of seeing children called "Thalidamiders," with virtually no arms or forearms but hands sticking out maybe a half dozen inches from their shoulders, caused the US congress to enact legislation to make the future of drug development much more difficult. This limited the ability of the pharmaceutical industry to succeed making new drugs available, including drugs for the mentally ill in need of all the help they can get!

Ethanol has been and will probably always be the most widely used calming agent. Salvatore P. Lucia, MD, formerly professor of preventive medicine and hematology at UCSF, famous for his intellect and his bedside manner was also a famed enologist. In one of his books titled, "Wine and Your Well Being," a glass of wine was highly recommended as a pleasant and effective sedative. There was nothing to suggest drinking a quart or two every day to drown your sorrows! The understanding of "fermentation," by the way, provided the very basis for organic chemistry, that all physicians nowadays including myself could use a lot more of! After all, the human body is a chemical system and shouldn't be looked upon like something assembled in an automotive factory. Granted the body runs on oxygen and glucose, however, beyond that it becomes a lot more complicated than an automobile or an airplane.

With all the problems "excessive use of alcohol has caused" and continues to cause, this visit to one of several wineries in Napa Valley during 2001 brought a surprise. While others raved on about "taste," nearly all wines I tasted didn't taste that good to me but I was not trained to be a judge of wine. One of the ladies offering a sample, curious about my line of work discovering I'm a neurologist asked, "Is mad cow disease a problem in the US?" "No, it isn't," I answered, "In fact it is not much of a problem in terms of disease threats around the world except for too much publicity affecting too many people's minds." It was a surprise why anyone serving a beverage every day that causes so many problems could be so worried about a rare albeit very intriguing "prion disease." True the prion disease that caused a mini epidemic of variant Creutzfeld-Jakob disease in England proved reason for alarm but alcoholism, a major social problem of mankind, has caused more mental derangement than any poor mad cow ever did.

Opposite to drugs that sedate, like barbiturates, that have been very useful in psychiatric medicine, are amphetamines. They have proven more effective central nervous system stimulants than their relative, an ancient Chinese herb alkaloid called ephedrine. Levo-amphetamine known as Benzedrine was used long before World War II. After World War II dextro-amphetamine, Dexedrine, was introduced and preferred over levo-form Benzedrine, having greater central stimulatory but less cardiovascular effects. Dexedrine, early on, was used to curb one's appetite. Interestingly a recreational "rave drug," Ecstasy, popularized in England beginning in 1988, was first synthesized by Merck in 1912! It was known then as an appetite suppressant, but the firm's decision was not to market it. Dexedrine, "one time favorite to relieve depression," proved useful also for treatment of narcolepsy. Paradoxically, Dexedrine was observed "to stimulate a calming effect in children who had not recovered completely from encephalitis."

Many persons took amphetamines in small doses for great lengths of time without any real difficulty, but the rule rather than the exception was development of "tolerance," or need for an increased dosage, to maintain that desired result. Not surprisingly "psychological habituation occurred," depressed feelings coming back trying to do without the amphetamine. By the nineteen sixties physicians were discouraged and afraid of being criticized over writing amphetamine prescriptions in view of well known wide spread "street drug" abuse over and above prescription drug abuse. Habitual excessive use of amphetamines, no question has caused psychotic states clinically consistent with schizophrenia. Users have been observed to see and hear things that are not there, indeed pretty sad.

Emil Kraeplin, first to identify schizophrenia, was the psychiatrist and neurological pathologist who credited Alois Alzheimer, founder of the German school of neuropathology, with precise pathological delineation of changes in the brain associated with "pre-senile dementia." "Pre-senile dementia was given his name, "Alzheimer's disease" by Kraeplin in 1907, commemorating Alzheimer's careful work finished by 1903.

"Alzheimer's disease was given a resurrection" by the nineteen eighties. This logically followed investigations using the electron microscope beginning in the early nineteen sixties. Pathological changes in brain tissue were studied in amazing detail in a variety of conditions. Due to such studies Alzheimer's name became commercialized into a "household word." Starting with about $250 in the bank millions of dollars have been raised. Well, there have been no laws I know of that make it "illegal" for neurologists, neurological pathologists, or Ph.D.s to become hustlers. Besides, even if it hasn't helped sick patients much yet, it increased employment, and with so many physicians and researchers that's very important! After all, if inquiring minds have not been able to find work, there's "no hope for meeting an on going challenge to figure and effectively treat disease; just don't expect results very soon."

Emil Kraeplin named his newly discovered mental illness, "Dementia Praecox," observing it often showed itself early in life, dementia later on. The name, "schizophrenia," was coined later on by Eugen Bleuler. Hallucinations and delusions, while common, were not observed as exclusive to schizophrenia per se. Bleuler gave us the accepted name, schizophrenia, and also his concept of the "four A's:" "affect," (dull), "ambivalence," difficulty "associating," and "autism," that by no means solves the problem.

Public interest in Alzheimer's Disease, as well as "autism" as a result of motion pictures has increased considerably. Movies have helped raise money for research, and to hire personnel to manage such difficult problems. The movie, "The Rain man," featured Dustin Hoffman playing more the role of an "idiot savant," managed for a very frustrating week by his brother played, also very well by Tom Cruise. Parents who have had mentally disturbed children, even one in the home (you quickly discover one is enough!), were understandably very entertained by that movie.

Schizophrenia is the only condition among the three, schizophrenia, autism and Alzheimer's disease, that can be treated with some success. Schizophrenia, also remits, and may for an interval not be too much of a management problem; that is until it exacerbates! When it exacerbates, especially "paranoid schizophrenia," the psychiatrist must be extremely "careful not to enter into the patient's psychosis!" "If the patient believes he is Jesus," you do not pat him on the back and say, "You don't really believe that do you?" If you do, you risk becoming an enemy of the patient! The patient remembers, later may obtain a gun and come to your office intending to shoot to kill. This is exactly what happened to me, however I was fortunate to have another psychiatrist telephone me as the patient verbalized in advance his intention to kill me, and reportedly was on his way.

Practicing medicine, like everything else, you live and learn. If you think there is no risk in "psychiatric medicine," think again! Not only is it possible you become the target of someone gone mad with a loaded revolver, you also have the problem of the woman, who thinks she's beautiful, and she is! She falls "in love" with you, next you fall "in love" with her! There's the potential for hanky-panky right on your office desk (!), thought of as "therapeutic" for her problem, and/or perhaps yours as well! Eventually the psychiatrist may learn there are more risks in the mental illness division of the medical profession than in "big game hunting." It's best to follow a set of iron clad rules, in which case you will not lose your medical license!

There is no cognitive gift associated with autism in the typical case or any case I have ever seen. The movie, "The Rain man," depicts something on the order of a "demented schizophrenic 'savant'," certainly not autism. On the other hand, the script contains some suggestion of autism. Autism is so tragic a subject to make a movie about it, and nothing else, would certainly fail to create public appeal. Dustin Hoffman and Tom Cruise succeeded in creating an interest in autism. Autistic children are reportedly not observed to have delusions or hallucinations. (Schizophrenics within my experience, do have delusions and hallucinations.)

Autistic children have impaired language development, are withdrawn, lack awareness and sensitivity and are unable to smile, bond, or even appreciate a hug! (That was brought out in the movie, The Rain Man.) One case of autism needed two years for the little boy to learn to get himself a drink of water, my role being one of helping hold the father together, as he determined with great patience to coach his son.

For treating schizophrenia the giant leap forward occurred in 1950 from French research. The French investigated a triple ringed anti histamine, promazine, with a nitrogen and sulfur atom positioned on its nucleus. The French researchers thought to add a chlorine atom to promazine's third ring introducing chlorpromazine. The French gave chlorpromazine the trade name, "Largactil," since the newly introduced drug had so many beneficial actions. Soon it was introduced and marketed in the US, under the famous trade name, Thorazine!

Thorazine comes in 10, 25, 50, 100 and 200 mg. sizes. It must be administered cautiously, to avoid a conceivable drop in blood pressure upon getting out of bed or up from a chair. Feeling your way along the drug proves to be quite safe in huge dosages (one schizophrenic patient I evaluated, from Stockton State Hospital, was taking 2400 mg. daily! exhibiting no obvious side effects). The drug in many cases helps to make delusions disappear (seeing or hearing something as something else), and also rids patients of hallucinations (seeing or hearing something when there's nothing). Disturbances of the thought process, agitation, and hostile tendencies are remarkably improved. Of additional interest, Thorazine is also very effective for nausea and vomiting, even intractable hiccups! Incredibly, the drug does not cause sedation! The shortcoming of Thorazine surrounds its failure to improve any capacity for experiencing pleasure or motivating patients to become more verbal. Are further structure modifications going to lead to improvements for these kinds of symptoms? The challenge remains to this day.

Continued research with three joined rings, "tricyclic structures," led to success treating patients with depression and "bed wetting" with introduction of imipramine, Tofranil, by Geigy Pharmaceuticals in 1959. The following year, 1960, Merck introduced a modification of the imipramine prototype, amitriptyline marketed as Elavil. Tofranil and Elavil became hugely successful, Elavil becoming the leader in the race for regulation of the wake-sleep cycle so essential for treatment of depression. These two medications, plus four or five structure modifications that followed, had many uses provided practitioners thought in terms of fundamentals of pharmacology of the nervous system and receptor site kinetics. For instance, these kinds of drugs proved useful for pain syndromes, tension headaches and migraine headaches as partial or add on treatment, and also for alleviating mild allergic symptoms, obviating in many cases a need for "expensive skin testing to identify specific common allergens."

Clinical experience reveals depression as the most frequent mental illness encountered. In psychiatric practice, perhaps 20% of the elderly are depressed. Judicious use of the tricyclic anti-depressant medicines make treatment of depression the most gratifying for the psychiatrist. Success, as a result of administering such medication, is measured by relief from guilt, apathy, hopelessness, loss of interest, preoccupation with death, as well as sadness to a point of incapacitation. Psychiatrists learn to be on guard, early on, during the drug dosage adjustment period. As the patient gathers more "energy," it's wise to make everyone aware of a temporary but increased likelihood suicide might be carried out.

In the forties and fifties it seemed enough to worry about one disease. Increasingly up to our year 2003, it has become common place to worry about several diseases coming on at the same time! Since the sixties, circulating cholesterol and the slightest elevation of blood pressure have become a focus of concern for many people. Physicians, properly taught, develop skills for allaying anxiety, but it has become much more of a challenge as a doctor competes with commercialism, especially television, along with advertising in newspapers and magazines regarding cancer, stroke, heart disease, diabetes, thyroid disturbances, allergies, osteoporosis and arthritis. Oddly enough sarcoidosis, cause unknown, has become a worry for some. Lyme disease, in the nineteen eighties, developed into a severe concern, even for those who hadn't come anywhere near a tick that holds the transmittable motile bacteria (spirochaetae) to cause it.

Dealing with patients on a close personal basis, explaining physiological symptoms from a "habit of hyperventilating," convincing patients their condition is nothing more than anxiety, sadly becomes something of the past. HMO prepaid plans offer their worried enrollees screening tests with nurses, not physicians, making follow up telephone calls to give the results." Tests that prove negative replace clinical contact" as a means to relieve worries about diseases. Radiologists, who fashion themselves as part of some technologically beneficial wave of the future, and who unwittingly often times cause more harm than good by instilling anxiety, call some of what they do "reality testing." They should analyze more carefully what really allays anxiety.

It's difficult to ignore a profession that uses a heading of "health care," that at the same time fosters a bombardment of advertised screening tests for the masses. People have no way of distinguishing the difference between good sound clinical medicine and commercialism. Many physicians trained during the past 20 years only know commercialism or quit complaining about it. Much anxiety over illness continues.

A television program known as "ER" helps convince patients many physicians of that "specialty" are "hot stuff," when, in fact, they deal systematically with problems beyond their expertise totally unaware of their shortcomings. The main function of the ER specialist, except for true emergencies, is financial. Such are urged to fill intensive care units (ICU) as full as possible whether the patient needs to be there or not. Nobody cares so long as money from insurance policies keeps rolling in. It's one thing to be able to handle knife and bullet wounds, and most contemporary drug abuse problems, but quite another to properly diagnose all conceivable presentations within an ER setting and have them taken care of properly. Some 45 million people in America are forced, for lack of funds or insurance, to obtain help in an emergency room rather than in a physician's office, the exact opposite of the way it should be. Psychiatric medicine is left out entirely.

Considering traumatic neuroses famed actor Charles Laughton, at age 19, was exposed to trench warfare in World War I. His biography included this letter to his aunt, not far away, just across the English Channel, saying he (Charles), if he survived, would never be the same again! President Franklin Delano Roosevelt, assistant secretary of the Navy during World War I, chose one time "Captain" Harry Truman as vice president. Captain Truman delivered canon fire in the muddy trenches of World War I leading up to the Battle of Verdun when 800,000 combatants were killed in six weeks nobody advancing more than 3000 yards! In Trumans' biography soldier Harry described WW I as "a time when the world had gone mad." Exposure to such extremes and surviving mentally and physically aided Laughton to become the great actor. The traumatic experiences of World War I helped President Truman face all the great uncertainty even under harsh criticism at home. In two terms Truman dealt with "more 'worries' per unit time" than possibly anyone of the 20th century," except Roosevelt, Churchill and Stalin. Think a minute, "the man of steel, Joe Stalin, tricked playing politics with Adolph Hitler, later with his Soviet Union nearly suffered a WW II 'meltdown'." (Hitler and Tojo came close to winning WW II! This fact should be instilled in everyone's mind as we face the future.)

As early as 1871 Da Costa described "soldier's heart" alluding to "nerves" and what was first termed "circulatory asthenia." The article was published in the American Journal of Medical Science. In was, however, Sigmund Freud who really got to work and explored psychological aspects whereby a patient's inner feelings were brought to the forefront. Such feelings consisted of fear, terror, panic as well as impending doom. By the time of WW I, Freud had it right, noting psychic factors led to physical symptoms. Soldier's fingers were "frozen on their rifle's trigger." The soldier was unable to fire the weapon, yet easily capable of moving fingers under other circumstances when removed from the trench.

Finally the physiological effects of over breathing at rest, or "habitually hyperventilating," from anxiety becomes defined. Breathing out too much carbon dioxide reduces the amount of carbon dioxide, the very "gas in one's blood stream," that permits capillary passages to be fully open at the level of the brain stem. With less carbon dioxide brain stem capillaries narrow, reducing brain stem oxygen delivery necessary for a person to feel normal. This causes abnormal frightening symptoms. Just sitting, standing or working quietly, patients experience physiological, not pathological, symptoms that vary among those having the experience such as: being off balance, as if being pulled to one side, numbness and tingling around the mouth, or, in one hand, a foot or one place or another. Hundreds of times patients (mine) are observed doing this. Pointing this out certainly simplifies the treatment of the problem by explaining the anxiety mechanism, enabling the patient to break the habit. Of course, it may be bad for "business." The normal relaxed breathing rate is about 16 breaths per minute. Watch it!

While a sudden explosion or bomb blast instantly suppresses insulin secretion, blood glucose going up from an alarm reaction, a gradual fall in blood glucose levels certainly can cause a number of physiological symptoms like hunger, yawning and sleepiness or inability to stay awake when you should be alert. In the absence of an important "detailed medical history" real symptoms, relating to anxiety and perhaps nothing more, are missed thousands of times. As a result thousands of unnecessary tests serve no more than to propagate, rather than abate, so many patients' difficulties constituting poor medical care.

For treatment of phobias, or irrational fear of certain activities, objects, places or situations, it is easiest to avoid such exposures, like snakes or spiders, probably learned as a child. A social phobia, like speaking before an audience, considered acquired before the age of 25, can be overcome with intensive coaching and reassurance over time.

For nonspecific anxieties like concerns over health, wealth, job performance, marital adjustments there are medicines reportedly useful such as buspirone, or "Buspar." It's worth a therapeutic trial without expecting miracles, but I've only seen it used on two patients and have no experience prescribing it. For obsessions and mounting anxiety, such anxiety relieved by a compulsive ritual, selective serotonin reuptake inhibitors (SSRIs) like fluoxetine or Prosac, or Zoloft, or Paxil are reportedly useful. On the other hand, the much less expensive but not exclusive serotonin reuptake inhibitor, amitriptyline or Elavil, the gold standard of antidepressant medications, 43 years after its introduction into therapeutics, also deserves a trial. Begin with a 10mg.dose, then feel your way along. For panic attacks, the 1959 Geigy drug, imipramine or Tofranil may help the panic and it should definitely be tried. For a mother, witnessing her child being struck down by an automobile diazepam, better known as Valium introduced in 1963, remains a very good choice! Why wouldn't sixties medications be just as effective now as when they were introduced? Something new may be different but not better.

For the jitters, not anxiety, many persons do not metabolize coffee well. A cup of black coffee raises blood sugar (glucose) by suppressing a factor that signals the liver, to signal the pancreas, to diminish insulin output. About half the US population are "slow acetylators," which means they metabolize caffeine, in coffee, much more slowly compared to the other half of the population that metabolize coffee quickly. Only common sense determines in which half one belongs. At UC Berkeley in 1952, a drama professor boasts drinking forty cups of coffee every day (four pots, each containing ten six ounce cups), and the good natured professor exhibits no jitters at all one might expect with fluctuations in blood sugar and "adrenalin reactively kicking in." He obviously is a very fast acetylator! Coffee, tea and chocolate, all three natural substances, consist of precisely the same molecular structure except coffee (caffeine) has three methyl (CH3) groups, tea (theophylline) has two, and chocolate (theobromine) has two, in different arrangements. Within the human body, methyl groups are donated (the amino acid methionine is a methyl group donor), and so you get some caffeine from tea, and some from chocolate as well. A little of each is nearly a daily habit for many. Moderation though seems wise.

There is no test that makes a diagnosis of mental illness. A psychiatrist must use his intellect and experience, and developed skill, to interrelate with the patient to make an accurate determination. As aforementioned, dealing with patients who are psychotic, psychiatrists must be very careful "not to enter into a patient's psychosis," tantamount to risk becoming a patient's target, particularly with a paranoid schizophrenic. For legal acceptance an examination is always necessary, but an observant psychiatrist can often tell whether a person is mentally disturbed by the look on the person's face. This is not to say it is possible to determine if the disturbance is the aftermath of being knocked unconscious, or representative of an intracranial space occupying lesion, or side effects from prescribed drugs, or drugs obtained on the street. It takes time as well as cleverness to gain rapport, and to be able to obtain the answers to important questions to make the correct diagnosis.

The differentiation between psychosis per se, and psychosis due to something identifiable causing it (an organic psychosis) can be tricky. My favorite example this elderly lady visits her trusted ENT doctor complaining she, of late, felt somewhat dizzy. Knowing the lady "had to have something," he quickly prescribes this newly released "patch" for seasickness to be put in place behind the patient's ear. It's a scopalamine patch! The physician soon afterwards must leave town because of a death in his immediate family. The grateful lady, soon feeling a little better, goes ahead and puts two more scopamine patches behind her ears thinking she might feel better yet!

The physician returned, within about ten days, to learn his nice lady patient had been hospitalized in the psychiatric unit as an acute psychosis! After brief clinical evaluations, and cranial computerized tomography along with routine drug screens, the cause of her psychosis had eluded everyone. Bewildered, her ENT physician went directly to the psychiatric ward to immediately check for patches behind the elderly lady's ears that no one of the psychiatric unit thought to do. In a brief instant the cause of her psychosis, scopalamine, was identified! Too much, of one of the oldest drugs in medicine had seeped through the skin behind her ear. Overdosing herself with this alkaloid (hyoscyamus niger: "Henbane," datura stramonium: "Jimsonweed," had caused her "organic brain syndrome."

Thousands of dollars had already been spent since nobody pulled back the patient's hair to have a look. The ENT physician, one time chief of the hospital staff, exclaimed to those on the psychiatric ward, "Don't you in this unit examine patients anymore?" A simple inspection requiring seconds was skipped in favor of high tech gadgetry. The CT scanner had just been put in place for the 100 bed hospital, and the chief administrator put out the word, "Use it now because it costs a lot to have such a machine right on the hospital premises!"

Was the scopalamine patch a "judicious prescription?" Maybe not, but so often with the elderly, physicians have learned time and again you nearly always must offer something! Very likely the elderly lady got dizzy because her pulse slowed. She panicked, and decided to visit a physician she liked and trusted. While the "patch" was not in retrospect the most ideal treatment, scopalamine was not going to slow her pulse further, in fact if anything quite the opposite.

The relatives of the nice lady who drove herself "mad" putting too many scopalamine patches behind her ears became upset learning about the unnecessary tests and cost! Why hadn't the ENT doctor told the patient to be careful and not use more than one patch? It was about money. Medicare reviewed the case and decided not to pay for some of the bills run up in the psychiatric ward. Just as the family had gotten close to their hopeful goal of inheritance, it had been further delayed. For awhile it was privately hoped the patient wasn't going to make it. Now she was, relatively speaking, fine again! Medicare refused to budge financially so a lawyer was contacted. Who was at fault anyway regarding the unnecessary tests, especially the cost of the CT scans? Over utilization so common why was Medicare targeting this hospital?

The lawyer felt he had a pretty good case. If this wasn't "negligence," then what was it? An action was filed. The hospital's legal team quickly began stonewalling, with a lengthy answer! They prepared to expand the verbiage into two volumes, if necessary. Ways were explored to establish new case law in California! The hospital's chief administrator wished he had never heard the words, "CT," or "scanner." He was blamed for encouraging the equipment be used whether it was necessary or not! As punishment, for suggesting something be done for nothing more than financial gain, he was about to be replaced to improve the image of the hospital! Perhaps the lawyer, hired by the children of the scopalamine victim, was confident he could convince the Medicare review team it was the fault of the chief administrator who ran the hospital. By the gesture of encouraging he be fired, Medicare might pay! The ENT specialist, now somewhat baffled and amazed that money does such funny things to people, began to understand why California has led the nation in physician suicides. "Screw it," he said, "I'm not jumping off some cliff at Dana Point to please some idiots!"

At the root of such a legal mess maybe it boiled down to a question whether psychiatrists might put down their pipes, get up from their chairs, and physically examine patients a little better! As a result of all the publicity all psychiatrists within 20 miles of Dana Point were probably asking their hippie male and female patients to pull back their hair to see if any patches were there. Some went even further and began to examine eye grounds and check patients for balance. Time invested was less than two minutes! Regardless, this new trend petered out.

Widespread over utilization of scanners in America corrupted the British health care system. American corporations, by very successfully exporting sophisticated technology, worked in concert with insurance carriers for the sale of expensive health care insurance plans to go along with privatization of high tech hospitals. On a train from Glasgow to Edinburgh in 1997 a prominent civil engineer with a son-in-law who is an orthopedist in Glasgow asked me, "What kind of disease would I have to get to use up a 1.5 million dollar health care policy?" "Neurological damage with loss of faculties from a severe head injury could do it," I said, "Think of the cost of all the serial scans!

By 2000 the US had succeeded in further corrupting the Canadians as well. American propaganda had always been steadfastly against the single payer (one simple insurance form) Canadian Plan. It was considered "healthier" to have a thousand, or even two thousand medical insurance plans, all in competition with one another no matter that the weaker plans could suddenly go bankrupt, leaving clients with no coverage, whatsoever. From hearsay "neutron Jack Welch," former CEO of General Electric, was never going to be satisfied until every Canadian physician had purchased a scanner using a "GE credit plan," either for use in the office, garage or on a truck in case of a house call. (How many credit cards does GE back in the U.S? 50? 75?

From our motor home we watched television from Fredericton, New Brunswick during late summer 2000. With Quebec holding out but finally giving in, those making decisions in all Canadian provinces had come to an agreement. Twenty three billion dollars was soon to be made available for improving Canadian health delivery! The needed financial boost just passed was going to make even more CT and MRI scanners available! Not one word was mentioned to encourage more time be spent for improved medical histories and better physical examinations! There was certainly no mention made to be sure to look behind patients' ears! There was nothing mentioned to help Canadian psychiatrists! It was all just a case of now being able to supply more and more high tech gadgets."

The best of trained psychiatrists, with years of experience, are put to task dealing with "personality disorders." Patients with disturbed personalities rarely seek psychiatric help. Typically the disturbed personality is convinced he or she is not disturbed at all, perhaps a little anxious but nothing else. It is the folks who are associated with the person with the personality disturbance that become convinced "somebody needs help," and it's not us. "Help," if possible, is going to be obtained by a psychiatrist, as neither a general practitioner nor an internist has the experience to properly handle this kind of presentation, or even a clue as to what best to do.

In the early fifties psychology courses at universities begged the question whether personality disorders, then called character disorders, were genetic or due to the way a child was raised. As a community neurologist, who for many years also evaluated psychiatric problems for the state of California, a clear answer to this question of fifty years ago has not yet, to the best of my knowledge, been formed. By now, however, I'd better have formed some kind of idea.

To reflect a little, progress in medicine comes very slowly, with some leaps and bounds along the way. In psychiatric texts, British physician, Thomas Sydenham, is on the medical records as first to identify a personality disorder. His description, published in 1682, states, "All is caprice loving without measure whom they will soon hate without reason ("splitting" is the modern term that describes such polarized feelings with no shades of gray.")

Adolph Meyer, neurologist and psychiatrist, early in the 20th century, had published the first clear description of "the paranoid personality." He separated the personality disorder from schizophrenia. Other observations, by Pinel of France, described a personality disturbance as, "Manie sans Delire." Prichard, of Scotland, preferred another way of describing a personality disturbance as, "Moral Insanity." Distinctive features of personality disorders were very gradually assembled and recognized over the past 75 years in the Western world and continue to be identified today with ten classifications now officially established.

Neuro pathologist Sigmund Freud (1856-1939) broke away from a study of pathological specimens obtained from the death house to change course entirely. He devoted his life to the challenge of understanding all forms of mental illness. Psychoanalysis originated with Sigmund Freud, who received his medical degree in Vienna in 1881. Following World War II, neo-Freudians countrywide were responsible for the narrow perspective in reference to Freud. Even high school students quipped about "oral" personalities (dependent and demanding), and "anal" personalities (rigid thought processes, prone to becoming obsessed). The term, "phallic personalities" has been less seldom heard, referring to shallow, mistrusting persons unable to form an intimate relationship).

Freud's experiences caused him to wonder if "sex" was on the mind of most people 90% of the time! That was what the neo-Freudians had to say. Supposedly it was this exaggerated emphasis on the matter of sex per se, that frightened Freud's former associates and friends away, especially Adler and Jung. Alfred Adler (1870-1937), a psychologist, distanced himself from Freud by 1911, to concentrate on his concept of social forces thought to cause, and correct, what he called the "inferiority complex." Carl Jung, a psychiatrist physician, like Freud (1875-1961), established a close relationship with Freud in 1907, then broke away by 1914, de emphasizing sex through his independent studies of unconscious mechanisms, thought to be underlying the cause of neuroses. Jung divided unconscious mechanisms into the "personal" and "collective unconsciousness." Jung also coined the very familiar terms: "introvert" and "extrovert" in his classification of personality types.

Neo- Freudians in particular were highly entertained by the efforts of gall wasp biologist, Alfred Kinsey (1894-1956). With financial support from major foundations, making it possible for thousands of subjects to be interviewed, published at last were the "Kinsey Reports" on sexual habits of the human male in 1948, then sexual habits of the human female by 1953. Preoccupation with "sex" by the fifties and sixties even reached grade school levels! Teachers, perhaps with "hidden problems of their own," proceeded to relate the results of these sex habit inquiries into the elementary school classrooms! Many children were much too young to even care. Some teachers got into serious trouble. One male teacher in Northern California, from Indiana, like Alfred Kinsey, lost his teaching job as a result and was never rehired. It was sad but he recovered, went into a supply business, proved to be a very excellent athletic coach leaving sex out of it.

Disorders of personality are brought out through interpersonal relationships. If you know someone who repeats the same mistakes over and over, never seems to learn not to repeat the same mistake, you are probably in touch then with a personality disorder. Jealousy may be involved and jealousy takes on strange forms. An apparently innocent victim of jealousy becomes a target. As relationships between people go completely wrong, the personality disorder successfully rationalizes his or her position and almost never accepts any blame. It's always the other person or what the other person did, or didn't do that's at fault. Seemingly blind to anyone else's needs, personality disorders are very aware of their needs and persistent to satisfy them.

People with orderly personalities desire to get along with others, want to be loved by those close to them. They respond to kindness, and caring, with some token of appreciation. People with orderly personalities learn from their mistakes, and make an effort to improve and not make that mistake again.

An orderly or normal personality, who marries or becomes intimate with a person who has a personality disorder, eventually faces and must try to cope with unpleasantness, distrust, suspicion, insecurity, insensitivity and lack of appreciation, or gets up enough gumption to get away! The normal personality wonders how certain people with disordered personalities get that way. How for instance can someone feel no empathy at all and be so quick to hurt those around them on almost a daily basis? When alcoholism becomes a problem it complicates the interpersonal relationship tremendously! Regardless, as that song goes, "Breaking Up Is Hard To Do!" This is especially true for women, trapped with children, who may for years endure a preposterous situation at home that sadly, but understandably and detrimentally affects those children, at least to some extent.

It is of course a matter of degree, the circumstances, and just how much you are able to tolerate before separating from a person who drives a wedge between you and your relatives or steadfastly drives others you enjoy associating with away. Oftentimes economic considerations keep people together who deserve another chance. Another chance might be another spouse, or another offspring! For a child who causes no significant problems at all, and who perhaps deserves another kind of parent, or parents, it is often too late for any reasonable adjustment.

Leaping from the frying pan into the fire becomes a big risk. Even opting for a better situation that turns out as hoped for, this still calls for an adjustment reaction that challenges the person choosing to make that change, to make that change successful as well as comfortable.

After some eighty years of collective evaluations, by the nineteen nineties, ten distinct types of personality disorders were agreed upon. In the eccentric category: "paranoid, schizoid and schizotypal personalities." In the dramatic category: "antisocial, histrionic (hysterical), narcissistic and borderline personalities." Last, comprising the anxious category: "avoidance, dependent and obsessive-compulsive type personalities." "Borderline personality" implies a number of features from any, or conceivably all, of the personality disorders. "Splitting," meaning love or hate, bathing too much or not at all, seeing everything black or white, no shades of gray, is typical of the borderline personality. This goes along with immense difficulty forming appropriate interpersonal relationships.

An obsessive-compulsive "disorder" (OCD) differs greatly from simply the perfectionism, obstinacy and orderliness of the obsessive-compulsive "personality." OCD refers to "severe obsessed feelings that cause overwhelming anxiety." This leads to "necessity" to perform some act to temporarily curb the anxiety buildup. "Dependency," as well as "passive aggressive tendencies," are common with OCD rather than oddly enough the orderliness and perfectionism of the obsessive-compulsive "personality trait." The terms are clear for communication between psychiatrists. This is extremely important. However, the terminology confuses the lay public since the "disorder" is so terribly different from the "trait." The reason is because it took decades and tens of thousands of evaluations to reliably arrive at such a distinction. Jack Nicholson, protagonist in his film, "As Good as it Gets," and "The Pledge," alludes to persons with OCD.

A passive-aggressive personality qualifies as an "eleventh personality disorder" by a number of psychiatrists. This describes the person who whines, procrastinates, dawdles, is discontent and complaining, but also argumentative with anger expressed indirectly. (Is the path leading towards alcoholic addiction part of this? What is your opinion, from what you have observed?)

To answer the big question, "Is a personality disorder, or personality type, of genetic origin?" the answer is obviously yes to quite an extent. One sees a toddler as outwardly full of fun and pretty sloppy. Her sister is not nearly so "extroverted," yet is extremely neat and orderly. None of this stems from parental influence nurturing the infant, the toddler or the child. Most assuredly it's "polygenic" (more than one gene involved, with bases sequencing a certain way on probably more than one chromosome.)

Genes acquire and lose methyl groups and inter relate with one another. Some genes are long and some short, from perhaps two million bases down to 2500 bases in sequence. There are just four bases but also a strict "base pairing rule," as a sort of spiraling "rope ladder" with a contribution of DNA from each parent is formed. "A"denine ties to "T"hymine and "C"ytosine joins with "G"uanine. A gene is felt to account for more than the expression of just one single protein or enzymatic action, and some 35,000 genes run the human body one way or another, not as many as expected prior to the actual completion of the two human genome projects.

The human genome project showing normal base sequencing and comprising all of the genes on all the chromosomes is an intellectual, computerized result of a "mathematically reliable guessing game." It's one thing to discover a "schizophrenia gene," a much longer base sequence than some short fragment consistently identifiable among clinically diagnosed schizophrenics, and quite another to make a case for a gene per se to be responsible for a personality disturbance. Schizophrenics cooperate, especially if helped with medication. People with personality disorders believe they are by and large okay until their behavior, judged by those involved in close relationships, is revealed and confirmed by others as not appropriate. Others around the disturbed personality easily discover that person is unable to evaluate his or herself as having some problem making them act the way they do. Any proposal for psychiatric help is usually rejected. Those who are judged by others as having a personality disturbance are not anxious to be evaluated. Only the most able psychiatrists are able to offer any real help anyway, and it's estimated some 20% of the population have personality disorders of variable degrees.

Nurturing, especially up to the age of eight years, most assuredly helps shape one's personality. Depending on genetic "susceptibility," either a normal personality becomes obvious versus a mild to moderate personality disorder. A severe personality disorder becomes unmanageable "Attitude," however is definitely taught. "Attitudes" are learned. Using intelligence and through more experience, relating with different kinds of people, and using common sense, can go a long way to help overcome an entrenched dislike for certain types of people, or situations, that do not ordinarily make sense. What becomes obvious is that there are way more good than bad people in the world of all kinds, colors and shapes. For getting along, politics and religion are considered two subjects best to avoid if at all possible. Why is that? Both are pretty much taught. Whether a person is "conservative" or "liberal" should not make enemies among normal personalities. "Acting out" or "splitting" in religious or political beliefs may cause problems dealing with borderline personalities. The separation of church and state is essential for religious tolerance. "Temperance," (Remember Plato) is of the utmost importance encountering different opinions.

Genetic susceptibility must be the greater influencing factor, otherwise how does one explain the troublesome infant, who becomes a troublesome toddler, who is unable to adjust to school activity? Often mother gets unjustifiably blamed by those not involved raising a certain child! By age 12 one's personality is pretty well formed, however the brain is not mature until about l6 years of age and thus a growing youngster is still prone to outside influences. How to best get along with the opposite sex is learned, suggestions welcomed hopefully, as well as for getting along with human beings of all shapes and sizes kinds around the world. With both parents working full time and too much television entertainment bordering sometimes on the asinine, the role of the teacher and the athletic coach, always crucial, becomes more important. Hugs and words of encouragement from parents take very little time and energy, and can mean a great deal! It's obvious. If dogs can be taught to become man's best friend, why can't children be taught similarly?

Once the "personality" is formed it seems to remain unchangeable. Think of the remarkable ordeal of one tough sailor, Scottish hero Alexander Selkirk (1676-1721), his biography published in 1829. It portrays a most unbelievable example to illustrate the human body and mind potentially can withstand a lot! Marooned four and one-half years on an island off Chili, surviving, "living like a wolf," before rescue by a British sailing vessel, Alex, believe it or not gets back to normal life! The bronze statue of him in Scotland reflects this. Statues are not erected for personality disorders. (Except when politics are involved.)

Protagonist Tom Hanks in the movie, "Castaway," survives acute as well as chronic disaster. Utilizing prayer, ingenuity, imagination (his only pal, "Wilson.") and "hope," he miraculously survives to luckily be rescued, eventually winds up "normal" again! His traumatic experience fails to alter his personality. It's quite a show!

As to the formation of psycho-sexual disorders inclusive of trans-sexualism, fetishism, pedophilia, exhibitionism, voyeurism, sexual masochism and sadism, the reasons, while buried somewhere in base sequences ("alleles") responsive to background experiences (who really "tells all" anyway?) becomes too complex and variable. People derive some pleasurable feelings being that way. "Why" is open to further investigation. Trying to explain, particularly subconscious mechanisms underlying, such peculiar activity must have proved very frustrating to Freud, Adler and Jung early in the 20th century. Frankly I don't understand much of it, or put another way, "The more you know, the more you don't know, and there is a lot more to learn."

Homosexuality, as of 1973, after a very great deal of consideration among psychiatrists, is no longer considered a disorder at all. What's the big deal? The American Indians let "their identified gay men of the tribe" remain in camp to protect the women while straight males risked life and limb hunting buffalo for survival. Many physicians, however, are troubled going along with this. Genetic based hypothalamus-pituitary-endocrine-system differences are demonstrable and discussed in scientific circles which seems irrelevant to the question of "getting along in society."

What are you going to do about it anyway? Who explains "love" or getting "lovesick?" If a man only "really" feels love from another man, or if a woman only experiences "love," from another woman, what in the world are you going to do about it? Ignoring factual information is not going to make facts go away, and people ought to have the freedom to live their lives as best they can. Life is too short to try to play it out otherwise. Isn't it best to work on achieving happiness as you are? Make the most of life. Do you know of a better alternative? If you do, what is it?

A treatment challenge, better still, nightmare situation apparently psychological and unknown to most, involves the matter of feeding infants, and those very early in development, who either cannot eat to survive or simply refuse to eat! Identifiable factors, anatomical and neurological, involving the motor system comprise a very small percentage! Among some 600 children treated at the Kennedy-Krieger Institute at any given time, amazingly with "team effort," methods develop that lead to success, but again emphasis is on persistent effort day after day! It's a case of "eat or die!" A "cure" is attainable, extremely gratifying when a normal eating pattern is at last achieved! It's expensive! It's difficult to find persons motivated, caring and able to even become involved in such a program.

The drug "Propulsid," in experienced hands, proved helpful by alleviating some of the psychological impact of dealing with these feeding problems! Regardless, both 10mg and 20mg tablets were taken off the market. Why? Propulsid was an effective potentially life saving drug but with dangerous cardiac side effect potential. Nevertheless it proved useful to those dealing with the life and death struggle to save some of these very young. Presumably (I'm guessing) deaths occurred, lawyers got involved and some huge award from the pharmaceutical firm was obtained. As a result, certain children among the group, who statistically would benefit from Propulsid, were denied its benefits and died. Some died anyway! Not having appreciated the overwhelming difficulty dealing with such problems there's that parent, or those parents, or somebody involved who simply expected too much.

Nowadays physicians and surgeons, who devote their lives to develop the skill to handle extremely challenging medical and surgical cases, may be exposed over some television channel as reckless narcissistic killers! Narcissism may involve, in part, not just "love of self" but fantasies one can perform tasks or feats, by watching, knowing or hearing of others who have done so successfully. You may think you can quarterback a football team but you really can't. You may think you can run a business successfully but you can't. After overestimating ability failure for the narcissistic personality disorder is not handled very well at all. This is rarely the case developing the needed skills in medicine.

It's called "the practice" of medicine. Physicians dedicated and persistent enough, eventually over time and with "practice," at last may succeed saving patients otherwise bound to die. A psychiatrist friend, focusing on psychiatric medicine, on more than one occasion handles a 300 pound paranoid schizophrenic, of American Indian extraction, who became extremely dangerous to others after a fifth of booze! It remains a mystery to me how he managed, and surely it was a mystery to him too! Perhaps the big galoot, drunk as can be, and suffering delusions, sees his psychiatrist as a "kind friend, in contrast to looking at me and "seeing a lion, jaws open, going for the neck!"

How does one tell if he or she is "normal?" Is there anyone who is perfectly normal? How do I know I'm normal? I don't except to say, "I feel normal." Do you feel normal? If not, are you willing and capable of doing anything to improve the way you feel about yourself? If not, well why not? Other persons, who feel good about themselves, are not going to help you feel good so what's the answer? See a psychiatrist. Chances are you're going to receive some assistance.

As a youngster I remember hearing, "Your body is the temple of the Lord." Abstracting, this is a hint to take care of yourself, always, as best you can. Are you doing that? Also I recall, "What you have in your head no one can take away from you." Abstracting, if you exercise your mind gaining knowledge in chemistry or music so as to be able to apply your chemistry, or perform as a musician, you may be able to live where you want to live, be appreciated, and feel good about yourself. You will be an asset in your chosen community.

Do you try to learn something every day? Do you discover yourself habitually putting others down to make yourself feel better? Many people do that. As a youngster I remember being told, "If you can't think of something good to say about someone best not say anything." Abstracting, this means accentuating the positive, doing away with the negative.

Why have a tatoo or a ring through your belly button, your ear or a nostril? Is it because you lack some ability to communicate in a less provocative way? If you dress like a slob, as "Tommy Hilfiger" provides all sorts of ways on how to look better, what sort of statement or impression are you making? Spending 20 days in Hong Kong, during 1999, people are observed dressing smartly and showing it! In downtown San Francisco, my home town, there are people preserving an interest in dressing smartly, but not near so many as in past years. Strolling through Manhattan, in Fall of 2000, dressed in a bisque (creamy beige) suit made in Hong Kong, it seems no body dresses up in New York City anymore, nor in London either! In Paris, late in March 2002, businessmen appear very well dressed. What's happening in America and "why the sloppy trend?"

Should everyone who applies to medical school, law school or a ministerial college have an official psychiatric examination? No! The overall problems facing society are not going to be better solved making things so complicated. What if the psychiatrist is the one with some degree of a personality disorder, then what? It is very much "a matter of degree," e.g. how severe is the personality disturbance and also about common sense! It is also important everyone realizes success completing medical school or law school, ministerial school or engineering school or business school is not a treatment for a personality disorder! In slang vernacular, "if you are a jerk going in, you are going to be an educated jerk coming out!

It's not the best situation to have a physician at your bedside trying to determine what kind of illness you have, and how to proceed, when it's obvious the doctor should have become an astronomer! It's not good to hire some lawyer, obsessed with righting the wrongs of mankind who integrates your grievance as part of his overall approach. It's not good to have a "reasonable judge" seated in one community and a "hanging judge" in another, hearing the exact same kind of federal case, rendering completely different sentences! Prisoners, comparing notes discover one of them got two years while another ten years for the same offense! It is not reasonable to have a black suspect scrutinized by an all white grand jury, leading to a trial by a petite jury of 12, eight on the petite jury black. Maintaining balance using common sense is essential for maintaining stability in society.

British philosopher John Locke opines all humans are born blanks. Most humans are good. A few, however, seem genetically programmed to become terrible sinners. Everyone must philosophically adjust to sin because there is always sin in the world. Hatred and prejudices though are taught. Luckily only a relatively small number of persons succumb to such teaching but it doesn't take very many to wreak havoc within any society. Mental illness is certainly very detrimental to society.

As a small part of four years of medical school but for three consecutive months during residency at UCSF I had experiences in psychiatric medicine at the Langley Porter Institute. Such exposure proved helpful and interesting, but hardly enough to make one a psychiatrist. It was by chance getting to know psychiatrist, Harold E. Day, founder of "Capistrano By The Sea Hospital (for the mentally ill)" in Dana Point California, in November 1964, that inspired me to learn more of this frustrating specialty.

As for Harold E. Day MD he was a "rocket scientist!" This wasn't a joke! He gave up his scholarship in higher mathematics at Princeton during the tenure of Albert Einstein. Harold would have brushed elbows with J. Robert Oppenheimer, who by 1947 was head of the Princeton Institute for Advanced Studies. Dr. Oppenheimer was the chief physicist of the

Manhattan Project of World War II.

Lucky for me, not being a "rocket scientist," I'd been a regional champion Olympic Games styled weight lifter from 1952 to 1962, so I was able to say to Dr. Day, "Look Harold, you're smarter than I am, but, I'm stronger than you are!" (Harold though was pretty strong as well.) We hit it off very well having some good laughs the first time we had lunch. Harold became my very best friend for about five consecutive years. Every time we got together I learned something. There was no escaping it and it was appreciated! He was a most astute psychiatric physician, able to size up a mentally disturbed person and decide what could be done in about 15 minutes. He also read EKGs, EEGs, studied pharmacology, and knew a lot of internal medicine from dealing with so many complicated cases from what turned into a huge practice. His specialty background formal training included four years psychiatry, and a year studying pathology of the nervous system.

Harold Day gave up mathematics, inspired to find out why his lovable grandfather, a locomotive engineer from a coal town in Pennsylvania, was rendered senseless following a blow to his skull from a dangling icy cable along a railroad track on the East coast. If anybody's mind was disturbed, Harold Day was dedicated to correcting the disturbance. He thus set his mathematical gift aside to learn as much as he could about the human brain, and about the "mind."

Harold was full of energy and very motivated. Establishing his own mental health hospital, however, caused him to be looked upon jealously, and in a way selfishly by those who just couldn't compete. Whatever Harold accomplished he did it on his own the "Smith Barney way," that is "he earned it!" Once I made a comment. "If I had a choice of 200 doctor friends, or Harold I'd take Harold!" Ours was a good professional association. He taught me a great deal about mental illness. I did what I could to help him and his hospital politically. In frustrating times, he never lost his sense of humor.

Dr. Day's only outside pursuit and real means of relaxation was flying. His first solo flight years before, he tipped one wing landing then the other wing came off and he came to a stop on the runway with no wings! Doggedly persistent, he saved up and bought a used twin engine Aero-commander, 6275X, from the Rozan Corporation of Newport Beach. During the time I flew with him, he became "instrument rated," got 98% on a three or four hour long exam he finished in little over an hour (typical for a "rocket scientist.") Flying with Harold to Monterey, Lake Tahoe, or Phoenix, at times caused me sweaty palms, especially near airports such as Long Beach and LAX with so many other planes flying around and watching Harold wearing his thick glasses. On the other hand, he apparently knew where and when to look, and flying his plane, "he was as relaxed as a baby rocking in a crib." He'd let me fly the plane, but corrected me as I had a habit of losing altitude. "Keep the nose up," he said. With all the political problems surrounding a facility for the treatment of mental illness in Orange County that Harold was about to face, "Harold was going to have to keep his chin up." I determined to help him do that, "free of charge!"

In 1965, the California Medical Association's "special investigating committee for mental health hospitals" evaluated Harold Day's "Capistrano By the Sea" facility, with 84 beds, and declared it was "perfect!" There was such praise, and absolutely no criticism! It was the perfect set up for treating really sick psychiatric patients. Harold, up at five A.M, together with his trusted nurse from Johns Hopkins'; they once made daily rounds properly taking care of the needs of as many as 50 psychotic patients! The care was efficient and superb.

This sixties situation was in sharp contrast to 15 years later when Capistrano By The Sea Hospital became the psychiatric teaching center for University of California Irvine medical center. At one point there were 117 psychiatrists on staff plus all kinds of other therapists taking care of just 120 patients, everyone bogged down with paper work! Called to consult you needed an appointment because the patient might be in the midst of "guitar therapy," or "walking the beach therapy." This gradual transformation, in part demanded by Blue Cross and other insurance carriers of California, proved so disappointing and frankly unbelievable there was no enjoyment being around the place!

Not a planned action, unwittingly Dr. Day's 84 beds accounted for "all the mental illness beds allowed then in South Orange County," according to the "Berkeley, California computer!" "Capistrano By The Sea Hospital," featured in a Los Angeles Sunday paper, back in 1962, as "the hospital of tomorrow," had an impact. It turned into a "threat to others in psychiatry." Regardless of all the praise, by investigating psychiatrists on behalf of California Medical Association (!), Harold Day's facility was boycotted! (For details relevant to the most seedy local political situation ever contrived refer please to: California legislative Hearing chaired by Frank Lanterman, (R) La Canada, spearheaded by Assemblyman John P. Quimby (D), Rialto, California, held December 8th, 1969, in Santa Ana California. There was a required quorum of six more California legislators, in addition to John P. Quimby, namely John Schmitz of Orange County, who played an instrumental role resolving the problems, after the hearing. There was also Leon Ralph (D) Los Angeles, and John Burton (D) of San Francisco. What an indictment!

Somehow Harold E. Day MD endured it all. He "turned the other cheek," absorbing character assassination, libel, slander, politically inspired public embarrassments, e.g., "he was once brilliant but now was over the hill," and that "he was "crazy," that he "ran a shock mill," and "he gouged patients." The fact his mental hospital record, only two suicides in thirteen years, was unmatched by any other facility in the U.S. was totally overlooked! "Six absolutely no substance lawsuits were drummed up by medical politicians, in tight with the Orange County Medical Association." Those lawsuits, prosecuted by a once disbarred Orange County attorney, caused Dr. Day's personal mal practice insurance to be canceled! (The "Baltimore computer's lights all 'lit up' to signal, what's this?") Provided "Dr.Day from then on did not enter his own hospital," the hospital per se coverage by Farmer's Insurance was left in force. A psychiatrist, George Prastka, very skilled and motivated, handled all the in-patients over the years until the six lawsuits were resolved, each and every one in Dr. Day's favor! Topping off the sordid goings on, there had been a $5000 "payoff" to the sub contractor who printed the yellow pages for the phone directory, to "omit the Capistrano By The Sea Hospital ad" that was in the yellow pages for 14 consecutive years! By so doing rumors circulated were verifiable by checking the current yellow pages to indicate, "Dr. Harold Day must have closed down and left town!" At the height of the success of the boycott, there were only three hospitalized in the 84bed facility! It was shameful, beyond imagination, to observe this considering the number of mentally ill that needed assistance, most of them not that many miles away. That was when I began work to get the "legislative hearing."

During these stressful times I enjoyed some of the best belly laughs with Harold Day. In my presence at least he somehow kept his great sense of humor. He didn't mean to be as abrasive with certain other doctors as sometimes he was. (At lunch sometimes I had to nudge him under the table!)

The best laugh (it was a killer) was during an appointment with the president of the National Medical Association (NMA-all black physicians). After Harold's sordid predicament was so carefully gone over, the president of the NMA said, and I quote, "I never heard of 'prejudice' like that!" In other words, here was a highly educated black physician, very aware of the not too distant past and those who endured "Jim Crow," and the "Ku Klux Klan!" (KKK), who came to the conclusion that Harold Day's boycott was worse yet! "Blacks had each other," he said, "But Dr. Day, you're completely isolated with just one physician friend (meaning me), since all but one other doctor, Dr Prastka, were fearful of even knowing you!" The president of the NMA lamented it was terrible for the community, particularly those who were mentally ill, that needed the help Harold E. Day and his facility could offer.

I wonder what Reverend Jesse Jackson would say if I whispered in his ear, "The worst 'prejudice' imaginable, is not about whites against blacks but rather "whites singling out and going against another white." Thinking a moment about it, Jesse Jackson would probably laugh and understand such a sad senseless saga about egos, fear of one physician making other physicians look bad, and of course money! Doesn't it make you wonder? Are the best people being selected for medical schools?

It seems for US society to survive well into the future, it comes down to "attitude." We must find ways to improve. Where mental illness is concerned psychiatrists of all people, instead of fighting one another like other physicians do, should be the ones to best understand the necessity of rising above this kind of behavior, letting who ever comes along that can handle things (mental illness) better, do it!

Samuel Clemens, known as "Mark Twain," a master American literary said, "Always do right as it will gratify a few people but absolutely astonish the rest."

In terms of "attitude" and "motivation" and what's actually going on as of now, 2003, it seems that we of the medical profession are continuing to fail to astonish enough people.

MEMBERS
ROBERT W. CROWN
VICE CHAIRMAN
WILLIAM T. BAGLEY
E. RICHARD BARNES
FRANK P. BELOTTI
CARL A. BRITSCHGI
JOHN L. BURTON
JOHN L. E. COLLIER
CHARLES J. CONRAD
PAULINE L. DAVIS
JAMES W. DENT
DON MULFORD
CARLEY V. PORTER
LEON RALPH
LEO J. RYAN
PETER F. SCHABARUM
VICTOR V. VEYSEY
CHARLES WARREN
GEORGE ZENOVICH

COORDINATOR
HAROLD H. GRIFFIN

COMMITTEE CONSULTANTS
DENNIS AMUNDSON
JOHN DROBNY
TOM KERR
TIM LESLIE

COMMITTEE SECRETARY
HELEN MYERS

Assembly
California Legislature

Committee on Ways and Means

STATE CAPITOL. ROOM 3120
445-8211

FRANK LANTERMAN
CHAIRMAN

INTERIM HEARING ON
SUBCOMMITTEE ON MENTAL HEALTH SERVICES
10:00 A.M. - DECEMBER 8, 1969 - SANTA ANA, CALIF.

A G E N D A

OPENING REMARKS BY CHAIRMAN FRANK LANTERMAN

WITNESSES:

Ted Thompson, M.D., Sacramento

Harold E. Day, M.D., Dana Point

Loran A. Norton, Managing Director
California Professional Guild, Santa Ana

William Beach, M.D.
Deputy Director, Division of Local Programs
Department of Mental Health

Herman Rannels, M.D.
Medical Director, Orange County Medical Center

Ernest Klatte, M.D., Program Chief
Community Mental Health Services

Mrs. Rosemary Saylor, Chairman
Mental Health Advisory Board

William Hirstein, Chairman
Orange County Board of Supervisors

G. W. Hawkins, M. D., President
Orange County Medical Association

Everett Bannister, M.D., Executive Director
Orange County Medical Association

Agenda - December 8, 1969
Page 2

Vincent Carroll, M.D.
   Southcoast Community Hospital

Robert A. Green, Executive Director.
   Mental Health Association

David Geddes, M.D.
   St. Joseph's Hospital

Arthur Jost,
   California Hospital Association

Robert Claar,
   Schizophrenia Foundation

Paul Grien, President
   Mental Health Association

George Scholl, Chairman
   Statewide Conference of Private Mental Health Facilities

California State Psychological Association
   Palo Alto

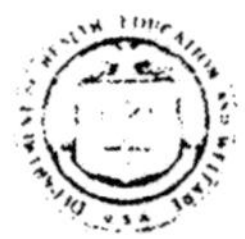

THE SECRETARY OF HEALTH, EDUCATION, AND WELFARE
WASHINGTON, D. C. 20201

2 6 MAR 1969

Dear Dr. Thompson:

Bill Callender has kept me up-to-date on the situation with
Capistrano By The Sea Hospital in Dana Point. I have at
hand your letter of February 20, asking that I call Thomas
Leavey of Farmer's Insurance and discuss insurance for
Harold E. Day, M.D., owner of Capistrano By The Sea Hospital.

It is my clear understanding that Bill Callender, in the
presence of Dr. Day and yourself, has already placed a call
to Thomas Leavey on my behalf, and discussed insurance for
the hospital. At that time the agreement was that Farmer's
would give 90 days interim insurance to the hospital and
that Dr. Day would use the time to find another company for
permanent insurance. It is my further understanding that
Farmer's is going out of the medical insurance business and
therefore, regardless of the merits of Capistrano By The
Sea, is not going to continue to be equipped to handle such
insurance cases.

I regret that Dr. Day has had serious problems with his
hospital and hope that all can be resolved on the local level
in the near future. I am sorry not to be of more help to
you at this time, but I feel that my office has done what it
can to help work something out between Dr. Day and Mr. Leavey.

With best wishes for every success with Capistrano By The Sea
Hospital.

Sincerely,

Robert H. Finch
Secretary

Dr. Ted Nolan Thompson, M.D.
5025 J Street, Suite 316
Sacramento, California 95819

UNIVERSITY OF CALIFORNIA
SAN FRANCISCO MEDICAL CENTER

BERKELEY · DAVIS · IRVINE · LOS ANGELES · RIVERSIDE · SAN DIEGO · SAN FRANCISCO 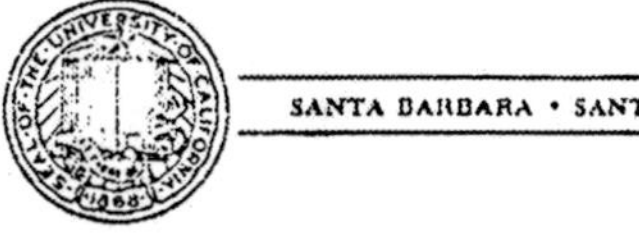 SANTA BARBARA · SANTA CRUZ

DEPARTMENT OF
THE HISTORY OF HEALTH SCIENCES

SAN FRANCISCO, CALIFORNIA   94122

December 9, 1969

Ted Nolan Thompson, M.D.
5025 J Street
Sacramento, California 95819

Dear Ted:

Many thanks for keeping me informed with regard to the problems you encountered down South. I am glad you have been able to stay with it and I hope you will keep me apprised of further developments.

With kind personal regards, and best wishes to you and yours for the Christmas Season,

Yours sincerely,

J. B. deC. M. Saunders, M.D.

S/dn

Salvatore Pablo Lucia, M.D.
350 Parnassus Avenue, Suite 601
San Francisco 94117
564-3520 24 Hours

Dec 4, 1969

Dear Ted,

Many thanks for your note. I hope that your pioneer work among warm regions a benefit for both thee and me.

Best regards and happy holidays.

Sal

CHAPTER VI

"SO MANY DRUGS AND SO LITTLE TIME"

The power of television affects societies worldwide. Without question there are many excellent programs as well as many beneficial programs. Perhaps one night a week should be dark. This would provide family members in each and every household a chance to think of something else to do.

My first awareness of something not quite right occurred during 2000. Interrupting a program that had created some interest came this commercial about a drug called "Zyban". The other name for the drug, "buproprion" brought to mind it had been released some ten years ago as an anti-depressant focusing on making more dopamine available in central nervous pathways, however it was not called "Zyban." Checking the physician desk reference (PDR) going back several years, sure enough, buproprion was released using the trade name, "Wellbutrin." As an epileptologist reviewing its' side effect profile similar say to fluoxetine, or "Prozac," there was an additional worrisome feature. In perhaps ten of 250 prescriptions, seizure symptoms were a side effect of buproprion (Wellbutrin). As a neurologist with a psychiatric sub-specialty, familiar with a number of medications already effective for depression, there was no desire on my part to try a new drug with albeit a small chance of provoking seizure symptoms. The goal after all of getting rid of seizure symptoms of various kinds a main stay of my practice!

Why the two advertised names for the very same medication? Zyban, a longer acting form of Wellbutin, targets the smoker of cigarettes who desires some assistance to quit the habit of smoking cigarettes. Why smokers become convinced they "need assistance" to quit the habit is somewhat mysterious since time after time smokers confess that they, after smoking two packs a day for 20 years, just quit! What seems essential for the smoker to quit is simply, "a good enough reason." If a girl whom a fellow who smokes wishes to marry doesn't smoke, and she insists he quit the habit, then love conquers all! He, in exchange for love, quits smoking. He needs no assistance, and that's all there is to it.

Nicotine provides an extremely interesting pharmacological study since it is extremely lethal in large dosages (as an oil it's used in chemical warfare.), yet quite beneficial in extremely minute amounts according to those who regularly smoke. Where the notion about nicotine's "being addictive" comes in is anyone's guess. People who enjoy smoking cigarettes and don't care to quit like to believe they are hooked. They use this to defend their habit, especially when others around them demand they quit because the secondary smoke is bothersome and more importantly is a worry. The non-smoker may be a "clean air advocate," in which case he or she better try some other planet. When the smoker is not so cordial a person interpersonal relationships with those around are going to run against the one who smokes. For instance if you had the pleasure of dining with "the great one, Jackie Gleason," would you ask him not to smoke?

Inhaling smoke from any colloidal source, whether it's in a garage or crowded highway or during a card game, is to some degree irritating to lung tissue. Only so much can be handled by one's lung system's protective white blood cells known as macrophages ("dust cells"). Fumes from industry, automobiles, melting plastics, forest fires and agricultural haze, all quite menacing, persons without optimally genetically well programmed lungs may suffer most as time goes on. Advantages versus disadvantages should be weighed in the balance. There are those vital statistics that indicate a smoker lives fewer years than a non-smoker. In the frequently touted "Framingham, Massachusetts study" it's estimated a smoker lives about seven years less than a person who does not smoke cigarettes. Asbestos dust is much more bothersome for the heavy smoker of cigarettes. Exposure to sugar cane dust is much more bothersome for the heavy smoker and, of course, so is a miner of coal. This goes for anyone who mines metal bearing minerals underground, or any substance under ground, challenging his lungs all the more if he smokes, thereby logically giving his lungs less chance to recover. The amount of lung tissue one has is another factor to consider, however, the volume of protective white cells may be proportional.

After listening to the television ad and a list of conceivable drug side effects rattled off in a whispering tone, the viewer is told to be sure to check with a physician and be careful not to take Zyban if you are already taking Wellbutrin! Shouldn't the person giving the pitch, in all honesty, tell the audience Zyban is simply a longer acting form of Wellbutrin and say watch out not to overdose yourself? Why don't they do that?

Reportedly one third of patients who take notice of such television commercials do ask a physician about the advertised drug. Busy doctors, tired and not likely having time to watch much television at day's end, are dependent upon patients to enlighten them about new products, instead of the other way around. Those involved in marketing pharmaceuticals are very aware of all this. Billions are spent on television advertising for pharmaceuticals. Those billions of course also support some very enjoyable programs.

The science of chemistry forms the very roots of pharmaceutical successes. Commercialism however, increasing over the past 20 years, has made money or "profit from sales" more important than "chemistry." One wonders how some of the advocates of "corporate America" got that way? It's not a very healthy trend. Instead of the physician gradually becoming familiar with a new medicine, and then cautiously advising his or her patient whether such is indicated, it has become a case of the patient, learning of a new product, telling their doctor they'd really like to give it a try! Some patients can hardly wait to try the new drug!

During the nineteen sixties and seventies it was a pleasure to spend 15 minutes or so with the "drug rep". With a twinkle in his eye, or sometimes just plain determination, he discussed the usefulness of his firms' medication. The drug representative looked forward to the physician's experience during a follow up visit a few months away. The usefulness of the new medicine was going to be decided by both physician and his or her patient(s). There was no pretense about having experience with a product the physician never used. The patient was informed of that. It was the patient's opinion that was important and the physician's position was to "listen to what the patient had to say!" More importantly, it was necessary to have a look at the patient after the patient became gradually adjusted to the proper dosage, meaning the dosage that reportedly seemed most beneficial, after beginning gradually.

Things have changed! Over the past two decades ladies have taken over sales of pharmaceutical products. At the hospital coffee shop it is mentioned last year she sold respiratory products to chest internists; this year the attractive lady, with great legs, was switched to selling "anti cancer pellets for implantation to thwart off virtually inoperable brain tumors!" After an intensive course held at the Hilton or Sheraton the pretty drug rep with nice gams has now been trained to "gam with a physician!" Neither the physician nor drug sales representative have any personal experience to base any judgment whether any good will come of the sale and subsequent use of the new product! If the physician has decided to date the drug rep, either because he or she is unmarried, or, the spouse is over in Europe, may God help the too many patients who are going to take this drug whether they need it or not!

"Nice legs" alone, however, do not sell pharmaceutical products! They do serve as a "lure" so that the male physician (most cases, supposedly) hears of the new drug. It is certain a physician will not suggest nor use a product unless, at the very least, he or she has heard about it. "Bait the hook well and the fish will bite," says Hamlet as he prepares to groom the players. Not only does the physician face the attractive lady drug rep as a lure, but additionally there is also going to be an on going bombardment of more new such products! It becomes frequently a situation where there is no time really for any doctor to gain experience with any proposed treatment before another comes along for the very same purpose!

It has now become a matter of still another extreme, because there was a time not too long ago when a successful breakthrough for a new drug treatment seemed hopeless. It took 35 years for example to discover a pharmaceutical improvement, for treatment of the epilepsies, with a product other than that great standby introduced about 1903, namely phenobarbital. In 1938 Merritt, Putnam and Schwab reported a new kind of anti-convulsant, and that year the Journal of the American Medical Association reported success with sodium diphenyl hydantoinate, trade name, "Dilantin" by H. Merritt and T. Putnam. Tracy Putnam, a neurosurgeon with pharmaceutical expertise, pioneered a new drug structure that finally worked. Neurologist Houston Merritt made the sale so there was "confidence spread everywhere for physicians to try the new product." Within just a matter of a few years the symptoms of epilepsy of various kind were 50% or more controlled with the combination of phenobarbital and Dilantin prescribed in good hands. This proved quite a jump from just 25% success using phenobarbital alone.

Physicians hailed the success of Merritt and Putnam as did many thousands of patients. Some time after, however, when Tracy Putnam thought to move from the East Coast to Orange County California, medical doctors in then this mostly osteopathically oriented area, failed to appreciate Tracy Putnam in "their territory." Conceivably their goal, of "preserving a necessary balance of mediocrity," was threatened.

Nobel laureate Bertrand Russell, British philosopher and mathematician, has referred to such goings on as the superior person "being chased by a pack of dogs." Have politicians at national, state and local medical levels thoroughly addressed this kind of behavior as of 2003?

Nowadays chemists using computers to visualize molecular structures might rapidly arrive at those necessary steps, to move or reattach a "radical" (a ring structure or two or more atoms that stays as a group), to hopefully make an improved drug that works with less side effects. Testing the newer molecule might be going on as previous versions are still being tested since the whole process takes 35 hours or 35 days, not 35 years!

Commercialism, increasing dramatically over the past 20 years, consists of "instilling a need for a medicine directly to any potential patient." The need instilled increases to become a concern that can translate into a worry! The idea is to sell a big profit making coated newly patented version of a drug to as many consumers as possible. Next, it's to delay the marketing of a much less expensive generic form when the patent expires.

"Magic bullets" or drugs fulfilling their purpose with little or no side effects are the dreams of pharmaceutical chemists. Granted, there's always room for improvement. However, it's absolutely true various newer products are either not better or not much better. Some newer drugs are not even as good as older much less expensive ones. Physicians more recently beginning practice are only familiar with newer agents. The US legal system is used to stonewall and frustrate competitors. Competition is delayed or conceivably eliminated prolonging a monopoly of the product. What do you do about a pharmaceutical cartel? They say, "If you can't beat 'em, join 'em," and some physicians on the "hospital educational lecture circuit," do just that while lamenting about the terrible state of affairs regarding medical care in America.

Free samples lead to paying for very expensive prescriptions. For people sold on the idea of keeping a watch on their circulating cholesterol level, only a reported 30% stay with such expensive prescriptions for more than one year! What good is that? How much benefit for a consumer is a drug that effectively slows the enzymatic production of cholesterol inside the cell, for just a year? By taking such medicine it does increase the number and/or sensitivity of cell surface cholesterol receptors, to incorporate more circulating cholesterol into the cell. What good is that for just a year? Patients simply cannot afford to keep shelling out the money! Business wise it makes no difference since if enough people take the drug for just a year that's big profit! Can anyone say this adds years to people's lives? It seems it only helps a small number of people, involved in "sales of the product," achieve higher incomes. That's good, I suppose, depending upon how you define what's "good."

Once a new drug is released and prescribed perfectly avoidable problems arise as patients are typically started on too high a dosage. The low dose responder is overlooked. Side effects may be severe from starting on too high a dose! Such tactics can also hurt the potential marketing success of a product. An example is the case of anticonvulsant drug Mysoline, referred to by internists who typically bungle their way treating the epilepsies, as "an expensive form of phenobarbital, thus why use it? Primidone is the generic, as good as the trade "Mysoline," provided the filler that holds the active ingredient is precisely the same as in the patented version as regards absorption in the stomach and the amount of active ingredient in one's circulation.

Pediatricians, in the nineteen sixties, ruined the reputation of Mysoline beginning dosages way too high! Why physicians have tended to prescribe many medicines this way has remained a mystery? The Physicians' Desk Reference (PDR) failed to emphasize the "very low dosage of Mysoline to start." The PDR failed to offer these instructions by 1960 and continued with this mistake through 2002! (Mysoline has not appeared for sale in the 2003 PDR.) As a result nearly all children (and adults as well) were bound to suffer avoidable nausea and dizziness as though overdosed!

My initial experiences with Mysoline were during a summer fellowship at UCSF sponsored by the Western Institute on Epilepsy in 1957. The beginning dosages used then with this relatively new drug were too high. The in-hospital cases just had to tough it out the first few days but at least they were in bed! Even during 1963, beginning community practice, the mistake continued starting Mysoline too high. One day, however, enthusiastic over success with the drug for the long haul, growing tired of persuading parents to bear with it and expect their child to miss a few days of school, it finally struck me, "What in the world was the big hurry?" From then on it was "start low and go slow" and let the patient, child or adult, adjust carefully to a remarkably successful five year stabilization plan for getting rid of seizure symptoms once and for all.

Using well-shaken Mysoline suspension (5cc=1 tsp.=250 mg.), a very low dosage to start or 12.5 mg. for infants and 25 mg. for toddlers, after the dinner meal did it. Very gingerly letting the parents raise the dosage nearly all side effects were avoided! Adults too were started on 50 mg. after dinner (2002 PDR: 100 to 125mg after dinner!) with the time necessary to eventually reach an effective dosage of 250 or 375 mg. every 12 hours being one week, and rarely a few months. Over 35 years of practice the highest dosage of Mysoline employed was 1500 mg. twice daily with no side effects at all! Another tactic learned with experience was extra folic acid be taken via daily salad greens, or B vitamins to make sure those taking anti-epileptic drugs (AEDs) were able to produce mature red blood cells. This avoided completely a not too common but disastrous dietary deficiency type of anemia that typically would be missed by other practitioners resulting in completely unnecessary hospitalization and evaluation.

For the neurologist there was nothing in this world more gratifying than helping patients get rid of their seizure symptoms! Failing to do so spelled a social tragedy for the seizure patient! Nothing more was ever required. Using Mysoline as the main stay and then when necessary, about 60% of the time, adding (gradually!) other drugs like Diamox, Tegretol, Celontin and Klonopin, seizure symptoms were gotten rid of 85%, or more. of the time for walk-in patients evaluated in community practice, a record never to be equaled by other neurologists trained a different way. Adding the second drug was considered when 500 mg. Mysoline twice daily continued short of the mark. During more than three decades of facing status epilepticus (mortality rates recorded as high as 40% in the nineteen fifties!), zero mortality and 100% success were both achieved using a naso-gastric tube for administration of two grams of well shaken Mysoline suspension needing to add Klonopin only on occasion. For status petit mal or "absence seizures" Tridione (no longer on the market) and Zarontin did the trick.

Under the heading "Backwardness Trend in Epilepsy Therapy," summarized on page 91 of "Epilepsia abstracts from the 22nd International Epilepsy Congress, Dublin, Ireland, Volume 38, Supplement 3, 1997," referees from 16 countries accepted my experience to share this information with other neurologists. Sadly the Meeting was so like a "trade show, emphasizing many of the newer drugs," my presentation was upstaged. Newer drugs had to be better! If they were not "better," why were they released? Sadly control of seizure symptoms of all kinds, in such patients susceptible to those symptoms countrywide, has deteriorated steadily since the nineteen seventies!

On 4/1/2000 a meeting was held concerning control of the epilepsies sponsored by the National Institute of Health, and chaired by Dr. Gerald Fischbach, director of the National Institute of Neurological Disorders and Stroke. Comments by Timothy Pedley, MD, chief of neurology at New York Columbia Presbyterian Medical Center, were mentioned in newspapers from coast to coast. Dr. Pedley was quoted, "We used to say that 80% of people with epilepsy could be satisfactorily controlled, but when you look back at people who are seizure-free, it's 20%, 30%, 50% and about 30% of patients experience side effects from drugs used to control their seizures." (It's almost unbelievable that Mysoline as of 2003 is no longer marketed in view of these comments.)

It must be emphasized that while the understanding of "why" seizure symptoms occur has vastly improved on a molecular and ion-channel level, success for controlling these seizures in patients, country wide, has dropped perhaps 50% compared to success in skilled hands during the nineteen sixties! Reasons for this trend include poor teaching, lack of experience, pharmacological confusion due to reclassification terminology, increasing vulnerability to marketing practices and widespread fear of lawsuits in the United States. Sociologically this has been a tragic turning of events of the past three decades; shameful for patients desperately in need of expertise for getting rid of their seizure symptoms.

At the Dublin International Epilepsy Meeting of 1997 one gentleman from Camaroon, an anthropologist was there to accept an award. He was unusually receptive of my poster and verbal presentation. It emphasized an inexpensive anti epileptic medicine, released in 1954, known as Mysoline as the best choice for a starter. In his equatorial African nation he, though not a physician, managed seizure disorders. He also stated his country was not able to afford newer drugs anyway! He gathered up printouts regarding my anti seizure tactics and experiences. As a result presumably seizure management now in Camaroon has surpassed the backwardness of anti convulsive treatment from teaching deficiencies in medical centers corrupted by the commercialism of corporate America. As has been said, "money talks."

Emphasis on technology, and bringing new expensive profit making drugs to market, has obviously crippled efforts to train neurologists for the one thing they should do best which is getting rid of seizure symptoms in patients they see! In no other area has the neurologist the opportunity to do so much good. Kids that have seizures in school have no friends. Adults that have seizures in public might just as well have leprosy.

In general however improvement in medical and surgical care comes along very slowly and periodically may wax and wane. The "practice" of medicine proves a constant challenge. Any leap of progress may be followed by the influence of many refusing, if not rejecting, any potential leap forward. All physicians are to some degree guilty of contributing to this situation. There seems no way to escape this stupidity. There seems no way to escape some widespread belief or fad that is in vogue.

Another variable that determines whether medical care improves or not is whether teaching exposures, within the many various teaching centers, proves as beneficial for one medical student, intern or resident as compared to another. While it's good to be creative, a physician mustn't be so creative so that other physicians are unable to sensibly follow his or her line of "creativity." On the other hand group decisions, whether "follow the leader" typical of committee decisions, or some plan to escape worries over malpractice suits, discourages individual physicians to apply their own teaching experience. If there are 24 cardiologists on a hospital staff it certainly isn't reasonable to assume all have been trained to think exactly the same way dealing with patients. One for instance may have wide experience with a certain medication that may be very beneficial in experienced hands. Because others have no experience with that certain medicine it shouldn't mean "none be allowed to use it" to maintain a kind of united front (defense).

Being a poor "committeeman," personally prone to dream of something else as a group rattles on about most topics, it is fascinating to witness a group listening to their "chosen messiah." For the epilepsies, referring to pharmaceutical products of the fifties and sixties, a "Dilantin messiah" is remembered well. The "Depekene messiah" is remembered in the seventies and eighties along with hype for "mono therapy" for seizure control. In other words what is most important is to use just one single product. But why one pill when it's just as easy for a patient to remember taking two pills as one? Well, "mono" means Depekene (Depakote) only, trade name for Abbott Labs' valproic acid or valproate on the shelf in Abbott labs for years before release to be touted suddenly as very special. Is it conceivable money from somewhere is influencing this trend? What committee decides to release a certain drug and why? Why aren't some drugs left on the shelf where, based on a great deal of experience in this area of expertise, they should remain so far as the epilepsies are concerned? Are favorable measurements in mice supposed to automatically translate into something terrific for humans?

With the exception of life saving emergencies and other rare situations, starting low and going slow, gradually raising the dosage of any medicine until it does its' job with the patient feeling comfortable constitutes "wisdom in therapeutics! " This is especially true with the elderly who like taking medicine(s) more than younger patients. Presumably many good drugs do less well in the market place because physicians fail to follow this practice. They start dosages too high rendering discouraged patients reeling with otherwise avoidable side effects. Again "Mysoline" tops the list of what can happen if something other than a very small dosage is used at the beginning. Another peculiar feature of Mysoline the very same patient starting with a tiny dosage eventually tolerates a huge dosage with no side effects whatsoever! Still needing to be learned, if the patient goes off a large dosage of the drug for just a very few days, you need to begin very slowly all over again! More yet to learn at least three weeks is required before any given dosage is maximally effective. "Therapeutics involves know how." "Know how" comes from experience. It is not a case of just anyone prescribing the same product getting the same result in the very same patient. Patients self-medicating may get into serious trouble. Pharmaceutical chemists succeeding with an excellent product must want to pull their hair out when they learn the product they developed is failing because it isn't being used in the most strategic way.

A Japanese mother in charge of all medicines taken in her household got two white tablets mixed up one morning. Mysoline 250mg, taken after breakfast by her daughter, was given to her professional bonsai-gardener husband! Orinase 500 mg. intended for him was given to her daughter. Her daughter managed her high school classes feeling "slightly different" with the type II diabetic medicine affecting her blood sugar level somewhat. Her dad became so dizzy and nauseated en route to his first job he was barely able to successfully drive home and crawl into bed! He thought he was sick with a terrible disease! He missed work for two days because of taking "one" 250mg. Mysoline tablet! His wife, frantic having discovered her mistake, related the incident to me by phone right away avoiding her husband being hospitalized unnecessarily.

Remembering this so vividly reminds me of comedian, Rodney Dangerfield doing his stand up comedy with emphasis on "no respect!" In this case it's "too much respect." The Japanese mother, her husband and daughter all subsequently enter my office waiting room, bowing most politely in the Japanese tradition. Father seriously wonders how his daughter tolerates such "powerful medication!" An explanation of the peculiarities of a certain medicine "Mysoline" turns the unpleasant experience for the family into a laughable situation as I bow in return. Many documented drug errors, however, are anything but laughable.

A UC Davis California student, who regularly "pumped iron" at the Sacramento YMCA, told me someone slipped a white tablet into his drink at a fraternity party while enjoying a few beers. He soon got so dizzy and nauseated he missed two days of class as well as one of his regular thrice weekly workouts at the "Y!" I asked, "Did you find out what that white tablet was?" He said, "Yes, it was a drug called Mysoline, 250 mg." The young fellow knew me only from the gym, so I mentioned "hearing somewhere Mysoline was one of those drugs that permits no alcohol taken whatsoever." As a neurologist, using Mysoline, no alcohol ever was always emphasized. Patients, without exception, were happy to comply. The most important goal shared was getting rid of all seizure symptoms! By eliminating alcohol meant preserving the medication level in the blood stream that prevented the attacks. Otherwise, as the alcohol is metabolized it inactivated the drug, in this example Mysoline, along with it, alcohol transformed by the liver cells into aldehyde. (CHOH to –CHO)

Potentially fatal side effects of certain medications may quite easily be avoided. This is accomplished by teaching the patient about the drug he or she is taking. The side effect can be suppression of production of a vital cellular element in the bone marrow. Proper questions asked during follow up visits include, "How's your 'energy' level?" (Red blood cells that live 120 days must carry enough oxygen or you'll obviously lose energy!) Another easy question, "Are you bruising easily?" (Blood platelets, one tenth the size of red blood cells, live 3-11 days carrying a "sticky factor" that helps prevent bleeding.) "Any sore throats not expectedly going away?" (Granulocytes, or multinuclear white cells in one's circulation, that fight bacteria, may be compromised within a matter of days on their way to zero production!) "Monthly blood counts for 'legal protection' are not really adequate warning." Bone marrow production may abruptly slow over hours or more likely over a few days! The offending factor, the drug (!), must be "suspected," always, because these clinical warning symptoms, or signs, may signify the drug needs to be stopped! The patient on the drug, educated to keep a watch out, suspects it since this has been emphasized repeatedly and without exception at every single follow up visit! There's a way of doing this, by the way, without scaring yourself or your patient. Regardless of what emergency arises, lawyers are kept away since your patient's medical records demonstrate how careful you have been taking care of your patient. Patients desperately are in need of certain medications. Certain medicines have great benefits and can be life saving and usually cause no significant side effects at all. Just keep everyone alert for surprises. Listen to your doctor. Be a good patient.

It is not common in my experience for Dilantin to provoke suppression of any element of one's bone marrow. Rarely it can do that. More uncommon yet (in my experience at least) is sluggishness for metabolizing Dilantin, or any drug at the normal expected rate. Instead of hours it can take days and rarely weeks for a drug to be metabolized and excreted after it's been discontinued. When both situations happen at the same time, and you find out the drug was given unnecessarily, it can become all the more of a senseless and potentially tragic situation.

That is exactly what occurred involving an exuberant 55year old salesman and producer of trade shows. Retrospectively he's mistakenly and unnecessarily given Dilantin in an Anaheim California ER. Having lost consciousness at a hotel bar he's transported to the Anaheim hospital ER, then hospitalized, paramedics unaware of events that preceded the patient's loss of consciousness with some muscular jerks. Why not ask a few questions of those that witnessed what happened or were associated with the salesman the previous few days? Why rush to conclusions? Why? That's what paramedics do! Or, is it a fact nowadays paramedics are afraid of getting involved for "legal reasons?" Or, are paramedics under orders to follow a strict protocol because of a city ordinance when common sense dictates otherwise?

Paramedics, of course, are not physicians. Like eagle scouts and tugboat captains with good training and experience, they are not expected to be physicians. Sadly, topping things off, many medical students taught over recent decades to be physicians are not "history and physical doctors" either! Nobody bothers nowadays, so it seems, to obtain some clues from a brief history of a present illness. What about "all" medicines being taken and, if someone who knows the victim is on the scene, a brief body system's review? This is particularly true of someone who passes out. This type event usually draws three police cars, two fire engines and a platoon of people standing around with nobody having even checked a pulse! Someone in the crowd shouts, "Maybe he's diabetic!" Such a comment is reasonable. In our Disneyland Hotel case, it's "epilepsy!" The ambulance speeds away, sirens going and with motorists pulling to the right!

The patient is on his way to an "ER!" Just like the television show a gurney blasts through swinging doors with everybody running, stethoscopes flopping around their necks; doctors all in a great rush with nurses holding tubes and IV bottles overhead. The exaggeration of an acute medical event, with failure to obtain pertinent facts leading to why the patient fell unconscious, is now on the verge of becoming a death sentence for the unsuspecting patient. Will unnecessary treatment kill the patient is the question?

It may be hard to believe but ignoring the recent medical history of any patient's illness can mean wrong treatment and, in some instances, "loss of life!" CTs and MRIs are of no diagnostic help. The "light bulb people," as bright as they may be, can't help you. "Charlie Chan" is of another age. "Number one sons" are unheard of the way physicians are trained today! What a commercialized defensive way to practice!

IV Dilantin is given in spite of the fact the patient no longer exhibits any seizure activity. It is anticipated, however, the patient is going to have more episodes of passing out thus he is "tested every which way," held captive three expensive hospital days. Extracting as much from the insurance carrier as hospital management dares, the patient is then discharged given phenobarbital 32mg. and Dilantin 100mg.by mouth three times daily. Topping things off, this hospitalized case lacking an accurate medical history as an example of mismanagement from start to finish, is informed upon discharge "his case 'legally' had to be made known to a state 'health' officer." Since it's "epilepsy" it's expected the patient will automatically lose his driving privileges! The patient is to locate a neurologist for what to do next.

The patient's wife is a registered nurse! It is a good thing. Unbeknownst to her, as well as her husband, in a matter of days she is to play a vital role in saving her husbands' life! Upon advice from other nurses in the area she brings her husband to my office. He's jocular in spite of the fact he doesn't look well. History reveals he worked to a level of exhaustion putting the trade show in Anaheim together. In spite of feeling very fatigued, he takes off for a day of surfing at Zuma Beach near Malibou California, getting wiped out several times in an effort to keep up with younger surfers. Before the opening day of the trade show he crashes for a very few hours sleep. Anxiously up early that morning for the opening, he begins celebrating with a "bloody Mary" on an empty stomach. Some minutes later he lapses and exhibits some involuntary jerks due to his "cerebral event" (gluco-neuro-penia), that results from a sudden drop in blood sugar (hypoglycemia)! There's no seizure symptom history whatsoever! There's nothing in his medical history to remotely suggest epilepsy. What transpired may happen to anybody, especially someone who likes to work hard, play hard and drink a little too much.

The phenobarbital was discontinued. Since he had been on Dilantin a couple weeks it was recommended tapered gradually with a 21day plan of two daily one week, then one a day for one week, then one every other day for three doses then none. (Sudden discontinuance of Dilantin has been known to provoke a seizure in a person that is not seizure prone! Dilantin, interestingly, has been given therapeutic trials for a number of other conditions.)

It was emphasized he absolutely discontinue alcohol altogether since it played a provocative role inciting his precipitous hypoglycemic event! Alcohol absorbed quickly in one's stomach, entering the portal system reaching the liver, is quickly converted into glucose. Should an abrupt and profound drop in blood glucose occur in anyone, it can result in a seizure. Blood sugar that has dropped suddenly and low enough (before one's adrenaline kicks in to raise it) may rarely lead to pulmonary edema and death! (Too much insulin administered for a diabetic for example.)

The patient's neurological examination was normal. Everything that happened was explained step by step. The patient reluctantly agreed not to use any form of alcohol and thus a good argument for reinstating his driving privileges was established. His wife was determined to make sure he would stop drinking completely. The patient said it was going to be awfully tough but he would quit. Follow up was scheduled for two weeks. With cooperation on all sides the chance of his driving privileges being reinstated were predictably excellent. There was, after all, a sound basis for a sensible report to a California driver improvement analyst (DIA). All that was essential was to explain what happened, what was accomplished, reasonably reassuring all concerned such an event would not happen again.

Within a couple days there occurred unanticipated phone calls from the patient. With each call he sounded "drunk!" His wife, however, said, "He's definitely not drinking!" "Look for a bottle under the bed," I said. More calls occurred. The patient sounded drunker yet, but both husband

and wife denied alcohol was in the picture! Later his wife telephoned to report her husband had a fever. "How high?" "Over 102!" "Are you sure he was not holding the thermometer close to a light bulb?" A couple hours later there was still another telephone call, his RN wife exclaiming, "Now his temperature's normal!" "What was all this craziness," I thought, getting irritated.

Was he sneaking booze? Was he playing tricks to show a fever? What was going on? His speech was really slurred! Was he faking and, if so, why would he do that? He was a very funny guy, but, it seemed inappropriate even for him (!) to joke about his condition. What was supposed to be so amusing about all this, to me his physician? Managing this developing situation became increasingly aggravating. What kind of case was this? He did sound "loaded." He, at face value, was experiencing spiking fevers!

The next day his RN wife called terrified! "What's the matter?" I asked. She said, "He's been hospitalized in San Clemente! With his temp elevation a local doctor, fearing pneumonia, ordered a chest x-ray but it was interpreted as normal. The doctor, however, has not seen him in the hospital. He saw him last evening when he got a blood count in his office that showed his white cell count to be low. The doctor suspected some virus then hospitalized him last night. Now the doctor has the flu and he's in bed, so sick himself he can't come to the hospital to see him!" I asked, "How does he look?" "His temp has been 103 and even higher! He looks sick, really very sick," she replied!

It 's not a virus!" "It's the Dilantin!", "What did you say?" she replies. "He'll die unless you do what I ask." "You must do it right now!" As a fellow physician, I cannot "ethically" interfere. Doctors don't call some hospital and order the discharge of a patient under someone else's care! In a way it's good for your husband his hospitalizing doctor is sick. This is some situation, because if your husband wasn't sneaking booze, "he's drunk from Dilantin!" The fact he sounds more and more drunk means he's having great difficulty metabolizing the Dilantin. The Dilantin, even one a day continues to accumulate in his system. His high temps off and on, that's the clue! A hectic fever pattern from a drug reaction! It must be the Dilantin! Forget the virus! Best you not mention our conversation so no one gets some urge to interfere! On your own, order your husband discharged immediately to my care at another facility. There is no time to handle this in any other way! Have an ambulance take him to Hoag Memorial Hospital in Newport Beach right now. I'll meet you within the hour at the ambulance entrance." "Okay," she said, "I'll do it! We'll be there! Thank you!"

I met both of them at the Hoag ambulance entrance. His temp was 105 (!) He looked red as a boiled Maine lobster! Immediately I ordered him placed in a laminar flow room on the eighth floor, where he was situated within an enclosure (bubble) of plastic, for protection against bacterial infection. (You can touch the patient but it's similar to what patrons do in Tokyo in those so-called, "Japanese feelie bars," meaning there's plastic between your hands and whomever or whatever you are touching.)

Unable to metabolize the Dilantin, except ever so slowly, he sounded very drunk and said, slurring his speech, "Doc, tell the hospital chief administrator I don't have any medical insurance! He'll send me out of here with an aspirin!" In the hallway his grief stricken wife overheard his comment, began to break down, seemingly sure her husband was a goner. "Well, now," I said, "If he dies he'll die laughing as nothing seems to rob him of his sense of humor. But, listen to me and trust what I'm about to say, and I'm not kidding, he'll make it!" "You rescued him! You got him here! You got him here in time (meaning hours) and he's now protected. He's going to be all right! Straighten up now."

From the nurses notes several specialists came in on the case. An "immunologist" and "pathologist" were unable to believe Dilantin alone was the explanation. As medical students we were all taught, "common things are common; uncommon things are uncommon." The infectious disease specialist that came in on the case was bewildered as well. Gradually, as word got 'round, it became the most talked about case in the hospital." It was a strange case indeed and someone called it "the case of the year."

Sure enough the patient, upon lab confirmation, proved to be extremely (!) slow for metabolizing Dilantin per se, (How rare can that be, one in 50,000, and who really knows?)) His bone marrow production of granulocytic white cells, (polymorphs), was suppressed downwards to not near enough to protect from bacteria to, finally, "zero!" The pathologist was alarmed! The patient, however, survived all the complications. His temp was held to less than 106 degrees from the time of admission. Bacteria, however, did find their way to cling to one of his heart valves and a prominent heart murmur (bruit) signaled a serious set back. But, IV antibiotics given in the hospital, then continued upon discharge-to-home, like Staphcillin IV, got rid of the bacteria and saved his heart valve(s) from becoming disfigured, and unable to snap shut normally; a fixable condition, but, oh, very expensive! His bill already had already amounted to $80,000!

The patient's wife, in on the case from the beginning, deserved a medal as well as a check from her husband's insurance carrier. Of course she was paid nothing. I made a few hundred bucks but more important than that, especially with all this disbelief over what happened, was being so tickled pink with the outcome. His insurance with the national association of plumbers paid the bill. Without that insurance they would have had to mortgage their home! I got his drivers' license back and the patient, last time I saw him, had returned to his jocular ways. Hopefully he improved his dietary habits, ate breakfast regularly, and minimized "booze," and important too, he'll refrain from driving himself to exhaustion in the future, get some rest before going surfing!

It's a curious thing insurance companies happily pay for a medical history when it comes to an insurance policy however, for the practicing physician, it seems insurance carriers pay for the most part for tests and procedures. Forgotten in practice nowadays is a good medical history. Why? I guess because insurance companies own the equipment they lease to hospitals. The hospitals as a result have big payment demands! It's all about "money" and being able to pay for all the impressive equipment, and maintaining that community "image."

A good medical history, believe me, is first and foremost for the welfare of any patient. Questioning the patient carefully for pertinent information paves the way for the best medical care. Nowadays, instead, there seems a minimum of dialogue in favor of test after test after test. One wonders how things got this way? It's important to find out what medicine patients are taking! For twenty years medical care becomes more obviously a high technology moneymaking affair, with hospitals packed with employees managing all that machinery. It shines and glitters as fundamental aspects of care are overlooked.

Obtaining lab values of blood elements by doing blood counts, first weekly then monthly when a patient starts out on a certain medication, "legally" protects both physician and pharmaceutical firm as well as the pharmacist from malpractice actions. However, this habit is no where near an equivalent of good medical practice. As in the Dilantin case there are other drugs that much more often may suppress production of granulocytic white blood cells in the bone marrow. "Educating the patient," without instilling any basis for panic, can mean a great deal to both physician and patient. Patients then protect themselves because, as a considerate physician you taught them how to do it. Should you not be readily available your patient, suspecting something's not right, will know what to think about, what to suspect and what to do. This is so important because, if you are out of town, you can't be sure any physician that covers for you will do the right thing for your patient, who may be on the verge of a medication side effect crisis.

Using Tridione (trimethadione) for "petit mal epilepsy" ("absence spells") consisting of drop attacks, (as kids hit the floor), often in conjunction with three per second muscle jerking and/or eye blink episodes), successfully and with luck over the years, a very rare and frightening side effect did once occur! Both parents became very understandably alarmed as a swelling in the neck of their daughter of nine years got bigger by the day!

Immediately they obtained consultation from one physician who suspected a branchial cleft cyst, then got another opinion from a physician who suspected a lymphoma! After that second opinion they came directly to my office standing in my waiting room, both parents and child, looking terribly grim! I looked at the little girl's neck in disbelief and said, "Stop the Tridione!" Her mother exclaimed, "You mean that's it!" "That's it," I said! Instead of a lawsuit I got a hug from the mother that might have made her husband jealous! Talk about relief!

Immediately Zarontin (ethosuximide), a multiple step structural variation resembling Tridione) was begun and the petit mal spells were all eliminated. The grotesque swelling in the little girls' neck, the most rare and bizarre side effect of Tridione, receded. Having never personally seen this before, of course I didn't warn the family about this rare side effect. If any physician, with detailed knowledge and experience pertaining to drugs and therapeutics within his or her province, outlined to each patient and family members directly involved every possible side effect, it's conceivable the practice of medicine, as we know it, would come to a halt! The herbalists and homeopaths rushing in to fill the void would, however, and without exception, get the surprise of their lives when they and their patients discover they have no remedies to offer for controlling, let alone eliminating, the symptoms of the epilepsies. (Never mind how the planets are positioned, or what certain tribal shamans use in some remote jungle, but thank you anyway!)

There have been idiosyncratic reactions to medications that not only engage great interest but also fascination. Again, the drug Dilantin has taken center stage! Famed stockbroker Jack Dreyfus made public his battle with depression that simply wasn't improving with psychotherapy. Someone suggested he try Dilantin! He did. Within a short time his depression improved, and Dilantin was given credit for helping him. The clearing of his depression was not considered coincidental even though many patients taking Dilantin, a drug released in 1938 as a leap forward in managing epilepsy, have presumably known depression as anyone of us might correctly guess.

By 1970 the "Dreyfus Medical Foundation" financed the publication of a book about the many uses of Dilantin. A copy of this fascinating treatise was sent free of charge to most all physicians in the US. The bibliography referred to over seven hundred papers covering the use of Dilantin for cardiac arrhythmias, neuromuscular disorders, sleep disturbances, migraine and other headaches, and neuralgias (peripheral nerve pain(s). It also covered how Dilantin seemed useful for disorders of thought, mood and behavior, even useful for asthma. Dilantin was also tried for pruritus ani (rectal itching)! On page 59 it emphasized blood element suppression from Dilantin was extremely rare.

In my experience Dilantin has not been a drug of choice for any condition. Nevertheless the book titled, "The Broad Range of Use of Diphenylhydantoin" has provided US physicians, who took an interest, with a fascinating read and it would be unreasonable not to consider it a contribution to therapeutics. The spirit behind the idea to relate this information to as many physicians, researchers and persons as possible was commendable, and certainly showed generosity and determination on the part of Jack Dreyfus. The treatise has continued to serve as a reminder many drugs designed for a specific purpose may have other uses! Many drugs do, provided the prescribing physician keeps his pharmacological thinking fundamental. (Why wouldn't a drug such as Elavil, an anti-depressant, be helpful for "pain," particularly causalgia or autonomic-sympathatic pain? It indirectly raises levels of two biogenic amines, including the precursor for adrenaline.)

When London born comedian (boxer) and actor Bob Hope played "Eddie Foy" in the movie production, "The Seven Foys" he also displayed some fancy, memorable, foot work! For those who remember that movie, the oldest of the seven Foys was Byron Foy. Byron Foy was the funniest and most amusing patient I ever had.

As head of "Eagle Lyon Studios" Byron Foy "knew everybody in Hollywood," and had special praise for Bob Hope, Ronald Reagan and, especially, John F. Kennedy (JFK). Byron was proud of the fact the studio he headed produced one movie in particular, "PT109". It was talked about at nearly every follow up. Byron admired JFK, in the movie the very confident ocean swimmer who saved nine men, along with himself, after the 80 foot "PT boat 109" was hit broadside and sunk by a Japanese destroyer.

Byron Foy didn't seek me out. I was the one and only practicing neurologist on the California coastline between Long Beach and San Diego from 1963 to 1966. During 1964 he came to me at the suggestion of one of his friends in Newport Beach. His regular physician was located 60 miles away in the San Fernando Valley.

There had been some kind of drug mix-up. Somehow Byron got hold of a prescription of Tridione. Excluding institutionalized cases Tridione was virtually never prescribed to anyone beyond 16 years of age! Idiosyncratically, Byron Foy felt "terrific" taking this medicine, an anticonvulsant designated exclusively for petit mal epilepsy in children! As a result he pressured his San Fernando Valley physician to prescribe Tridione for him! The doctor nervously wrote the prescription asking that he promise (!) to seek out a neurologist!

Byron Foy had no reason to ask that I prescribe Tridione. He already had refill authorizations and as many Tridione capsules as he felt he needed! My job was to try to explain the mystery of why it was so beneficial (for him!). In terms of the drug's side effect profile alone, no peer review team of physicians would dream of approving a prescription of Tridione for any adult, let alone someone over fifty!

In defense of the San Fernando Valley prescribing doctor, caught up in this therapeutic predicament, it was nonetheless understandable for the doctor to risk facing criticism, even if it meant the Board of Medical Examiners! What was a physician supposed to do if someone known as "Big Tuna" from Chicago; someone who runs a string of pizza parlors, along with other activities, telephones and says, "Doctor, I am 'asking' you to do Byron Foy a favor. I thank you in advance for doing this favor. Thank you again!" (click) For those of you who have somehow failed to comprehend the meaning of "playing the percentages" you could write to Francis Ford Coppola at his home (and vineyard) at Napa Valley, California, so his secretary can send you a "printout" with a very simple but important explanation..

"Byron, you feel 'good' taking Tridione?" I asked. He said, "I feel 'great' taking it!" "It's a prescription reserved for children and young teenagers." "Maybe that's it, I feel like a 'kid' taking it," was his reply. Byron Foy liked Tridione! There seemed no way to talk him out of it. He felt so good taking it why shouldn't he keep taking it? What was I supposed to say, "You can't feel good taking it, it's impossible? "

Byron kept regular visits. Each time I reiterated Tridione was intended for seizure symptoms that occur in infants, toddlers and children, not adults! It was a drug intended to prevent vacant spells and involuntary body jerks, caused by repeated electrical discharges from the depths of the brain, each lasting a third of a second but often occurring in brief clusters with a cluster lasting a few seconds. I explained to Byron that Tridione was effective for preventing attacks consisting of a sudden inability to oppose gravity. Toddlers instantaneously just fall to the floor! It's a phenomenon timed with a burst of three per second spike and slow brain wave activity. "Byron, I said, "there's nothing in your history to remotely suggest such symptoms!" Byron didn't care. He listened and smiled and, with a twinkle in his eye, typically changed the subject. He obviously liked having some fun with me.

Once I abruptly changed the subject and asked Byron Foy, "What do you think of Laura Devon?" (She was a young actress in a sixties television show featuring dolphins). He said, "I'll get 'you' a date with her!" In a flash he reached across my desk and grabbed my telephone. He quickly dialed some number asking, "Where's Laura Devon. I have a doctor friend of mine that wants a date with her!" His conversation, with some pauses, lasted about a minute. He hung up and said, "I'll get you a date with her, but it will have to wait because, right now, she's in Florida!" For Byron, maybe the Tridione was working like an "upper!" Its' benefit for him was idiosyncratic (a "feel good capsule") with no benefits documented otherwise. After all, he began taking it by pure accident! In a few months Byron Foy stopped coming in. Last word heard on the whereabouts of Laura Devon she was still in Florida. Byron returned to Chicago, I guess. I knew he had business there. It was ten years later or so I learned Newport Beach internist, John ("Jack") Skinner had hospitalized Byron Foy at Hoag Memorial Hospital. Jack told me Byron was on the phone almost constantly, while in the hospital, mostly talking to somebody in Florida! No doubt he kept Doctor Skinner and all the nurses very entertained. I specifically asked what medicines he was taking. Tridione wasn't one of them. Byron Foy, a most entertaining personality, I was told passed away sometime in the mid-nineteen seventies and he is missed.

For possibly two decades there has been an increasing trend to seek evaluation in emergency rooms rather than in physician's offices. This has been in concert with a growing trend of unnecessary tests, unnecessary prescriptions, over utilization, unnecessary hospitalizations along with diagnoses that turned out to be simply incorrect.

In May 2000 an 18year old daughter, of a long time friend's girl friend, was seen in an ER in Cincinnati, Ohio. She presented with a splitting headache and a stiff neck! Perhaps the docs were tired and overworked. In the fifties 8 hour shifts were common but in recent decades it became "shifts of 24hours!" Instead of keeping her for observation, she was sent home with a diagnosis of migraine headache. No spinal fluid examination was obtained to exclude meningitis, or a sub-arachnoid hemorrhage, perhaps due to a ruptured berry aneurysm, or to see if her cerebral spinal fluid pressure happened to be elevated! More strange yet, she "had insurance coverage!" Regardless, nothing more was done. She toughed it out for several days until at last she was evaluated by a neurologist. He reportedly obtained clear spinal fluid and labeled her condition "aseptic meningitis." Decadron reasonably could have helped her terrible headache had she been handled more thoughtfully when first seen in the ER. No medication was given to her at all, according to related information. Happily, though she suffered, she got better on her own. The ER doctors were lucky.

In a less hectic office setting her case may have turned out representing something entirely different like a breaking out of herpes II virus. From hypersensitivity to the activated herpes virus brain swelling may have accounted for her awful headache. Her stiff neck, if indeed it was as stiff as I was told, was a signal to obtain spinal fluid studies. In the ER the spinal tap was omitted and no medicine was even offered for her headache.

Many presentations demand wider experience, and a little more time for clear thinking, not always obtainable in busy emergency rooms where knife and bullet traumas and street drug abuses are the norm. Is it unreasonable to wonder if good medical care, in general, is becoming increasingly short of the mark as we begin the next century?

For psychiatric medicine it's disappointing to learn haloperidol or Haldol is prescribed so often for mentally ill. A most powerful central nervous system dopamine receptor blocker, it renders many "Parkinsonian," with extreme slowness or poverty of muscle movements (dystonia), drooling, and a mask like facial expression. Except for akathisia from the drug, whereby the patient simply can't sit still and exhibits quivering and motor restlessness, Haldol's side effects are likened by some to a "pharmacological straight jacket." Mentally ill relate to such a fear of being given Haldol it prevents their seeking help at mental health facilities! They know from experience they will likely be given this drug or something similar and suffer, without renewed evaluation, since a computer record of a previous impression is quickly viewed. Who's going to challenge what's on the computer screen? Typically Haldol is administered with Cogentin, indirectly intended to reduce the impact of such clinically evident side effects via balancing the blocked effect of dopamine by Haldol. Remembering past Haldol experiences as terrifying many that need help collectively choose to remain in the streets. It's a case of prospective mentally ill patients being wiser than those offering too standardized prescriptions at least in some facilities.

It's not just Haldol The beat goes on! In 2002 there are cases where general practitioners, and part time ER physicians, prescribe relatively new drugs like Olanzapine marketed as an anti schizophrenic, anti "Alzheimer," anti "bipolar" drug with the trade name, Zyprexa. It's no small wonder it's a best seller! It flies off the shelf.

Zyprexa is a best seller because inexperienced doctors prescribe it. They are unable to diagnose the patients that get the drug. Like indiscriminate use of antibiotics, it's just "shot gun therapy." Prescribing a sophisticated anti psychotic agent such as Zyprexa, that predictably blocks serotonin and dopamine nerve network receptors is beyond the expertise of all but able psychiatrists. Who keeps watch on the patient? Who knows what to look for and is able to judge the real benefits of such medication? Zyprexa is a big seller because a prescription for Zyprexa may be written by any licensed MD whether he or she knows anything about psychiatric medicine or not. For elderly in convalescent homes it's nothing more than a high priced prescription to "control a patient." Disruptive behavior is commonly due to the influence of a troublesome roommate and nothing more, not even requiring a prescription. It's all very sad, but good for "business."

Only a good psychiatrist knows if a mentally disturbed patient represents agitated depression, or a borderline personality, or an organic psychosis from a drug, or too much alcohol for too long. Statistically it's unlikely the patient has plaques, tangles and typical fibrillary changes in his or her brain's neurons constituting Alzheimer's disease. Radiological studies, by the way, may reveal some apparent atrophy of the brain that may have no clinical significance at all. Diagnosis remains unknown. Space-occupying lesions are ruled out. What's the answer when unnecessary prescriptions are given? Complain to a drug company? Is a drug firm supposed to campaign or advertise to please use one of its products less often? A drug for schizophrenics is used indiscriminately. Who's to blame? Is it physician training, or too aggressive salesmanship from certain pharmaceutical firms? What's the answer?

Discontinuing even a short run with Haldol or Zyprexa, as the "new and improved agent," may pose an unhappy risk of tardive dyskinesia, more so by my observations, than kinder dopamine blocking drugs intended to alleviate psychotic states. There is no predictable successful treatment for tardive dyskinesia. It only rarely gets better on its own. Because of grotesque involuntary facial distortions, typically a continuance of a milder similar drug is necessary to bring the undesirable facial movements under control! Whether the drug or one similar to it proved effective at all for the mental illness is forgotten. Needless to say such therapeutic dilemmas get very discouraging and test the best psychiatrist. Do you think general practitioners and emergency room physicians are the ones to involve themselves in these situations? Isn't it better to know a little bit about what you are doing?

From Belgian research in anesthesia in the fifties Haldol comes along. Like anesthetics it can rarely cause malignant hyperthermia. This consists of a very rapid rise in body temperature that needs to be treated very quickly with heroic cooling measures, otherwise it's fatal. Incidently, malignant hyperthermia remains still another underestimated risk with Phencyclidine, the veterinary anesthetic sold on the streets as 'Angel Dust," with a high degree of unpredictability.

Ecstasy encourages serotonin to be "gradually released by certain brain cells" and expectedly elevate one's temperature. Serotonin is the body's heat producing chemical of the nervous and endocrine systems. Serotonin opposes the body's cooling chemical, another biogenic amine called nor-adrenaline. ("nor" means without a methyl group)

Angel Dust, or PCP, may trick managing observers in a drug abuse case by lowering body temperature just before the patient suddenly overheats (and dies) if nobody is close by to anticipate and be alert to what's happening. Similar situations no doubt can occur with Ketamine, an anesthetic patented by Parke Davis in 1966, popularly used as a form of contemporary drug abuse called "tripping" as it is snorted or ingested.

Interestingly very tiny doses of Haldol have proven useful and, oddly enough, frankly helpful for control of the abnormal involuntary movements and the fowl expletive utterances of the Gilles de la Tourette syndrome. Once again it has been the very small dose that has helped instead of a large dosage that upsets the therapeutic benefit.

Thorazine, the great anti psychotic breakthrough, has remained available to this day. In the nineteen fifties, sixties and most of the seventies it was the most frequently used anti psychotic medicine, and rightly so. Thorazine has been safely given in whopping dosages as long as it is started low to avoid a drop of one's blood pressure upon standing up while the patient adjusts to a steady state of the medicine.

During 1980 or close enough nearly all, if not all, of the mental health units in Orange County California switched from Thorazine to Haldol and Navane! How it happened was amazing, sudden and bewildering. As if a Pied Piper had come through town, a dynamic psychiatrist from the East Coast hyped Haldol and Navane and the newer therapeutic approach took hold. It didn't seem to matter whether a schizophrenic was agitated or apathetic. The psychiatrist's persuasive presentations in area hospitals proved succinct and overwhelming in favor of the need for a "change!" If, as suspected, this psychiatrist happened to be on a drug firm's payroll it was a cinch they were paying for one good salesman! Working for a paint company he would have repeatedly been "salesman of the year!" Haldol and Navane, however, were not products to be applied with a brush, and any sinful results of such a sudden switch in drug policy remain to this day unknown. Those having routinely prescribed Haldol and Navane today likely have not ever used Thorazine. Probably too few psychiatrists today have had wide enough experience to know the difference.

During 1998 it came to my attention that Pfizer had developed quite an effective sales force. In response to a casual friend's question, "Doc, am I taking too many drugs," I investigated. Cardura was one, used to relax prostate and bladder neck muscles. Procardia was another for reducing blood pressure via dilation of the arterial system. He was on five medications. Checking the PDR, four of them were Pfizer drugs! When I called him, as requested, his wife answered. Hearing the news, she blurted, "I knew it, I knew it!" Two months later he was under care of another cardiologist. His medication load was reduced to two medicines. We crossed paths again in January 2001 and the fellow looked happier. As a retired electrical engineer from MacDonnell-Douglas, he had more electrical work on yachts in the harbor than he could handle. Smiling he asked how I was doing, and made no mention of medications at all. Two drugs proved better than five. Both he and his wife suspected he had been taking too much medication all during the mid-nineteen nineties and apparently he was.

By the nineteen nineties there developed so much mistrust and dissatisfaction among people seeking medical care it was common and not unreasonable to be asked to respond to comments about proposed procedures or drugs. Casually questions came from acquaintances that know you simply as "Doc," when you run across someone taking a walk.

Antibiotics have probably always been used much too often and unnecessarily, but occasionally they are necessary and by all means "indicated!" Taking a stroll a lady introduced me to her daughter visiting from Idaho. She then said, "Look at my forearm where a dog bit me a couple days ago puncturing the skin. My daughter has been putting warm compresses on the wound." I startled at red streaks proceeding up her arm and asked, "Where are you parked?" "Do you have a medical plan?" "Kaiser?" "Perfect!" Observing and knowing a little about streptococcal bacteria, I said, "Please get going right now and no more warm compresses! It's a 30 minute drive!" About a week later she thanked me. The physician at Kaiser was reportedly very happy for the opportunity to treat her wound in time and administer appropriate antibiotics. Flesh eating bacteria like streptococcus pyogenes that also cause "cellulitis" have proven to be serious and costly problems. Infectious disease experts respond very quickly.

Life is too short not to own some kind of boat. You get to know people you would otherwise never have a chance to meet. Angelman ketches built at "Wilbo" in Wilmington, California are my chosen favorites. In the slip next to mine at Dana Point California comes a new arrival for 90 days. Aboard there is a pleasant fellow preparing his forty footer for an expensive trip through the Panama Canal. Verbal and motor responses are hesitant and his speech is slurred. Observing that, it seems amazing to me he got the boat so nicely in the slip. A couple weeks later I notice a pretty gal in her twenties on board. She relates that she and her sister, and her dad, are getting ready to sail their boat, via Panama, into the Caribbean. "Are you a good sailor," I ask? "Pretty good," she replies. Privately, I'm wondering if she pays close attention to her dad, especially the slowness of his speech and the way he moved so slowly just days before. There's wonderment how the three of them are so frankly "enthusiastic" about making this difficult voyage. San Francisco to Cabo San Lucas constitutes my sailing experience(s) of the past 40 years. California and Mexican "coastal" sailing, however, separates the men from the boys. Panama is over three times as far as Cabo. It's a challenge, and no honest sober person with such experience, particularly sailing day and night, would downplay it. Maybe time is not a factor. They'll take their time and cautiously creep along. The whole idea of just two young girls and their dad, with a "condition," sailing off to Panama in a forty-foot knockabout sailboat definitely engages my attention.

Some two weeks later her dad, the "captain," approaches me, "Someone at the dock told me you're a neurologist." I said, "Yes, that's right." He said, "I'm a physician too. Would you please have a look at my most recent MRI?" His name is Jack. Together we look at his magnetic resonance images. Jack points to the former location of his grade II (or III) astrocytoma, a brain tumor, removed some 12 years ago. "Guess they 'got it all' (how would anyone know?), since I am still here!" he said. "Say, how much do you think my monthly drug bill is?" "$300.per month!" I ask, "What drugs are you taking and why?" "felbamate (Felbatol) and gabapentin (Neurontin)," he replies. He's taking both in very large doses out of fear of seizures instilled in him since his surgery. His anti-convulsants are routine post brain surgery, not because he ever actually had any known spells! Both are new touted drugs of recent years, both expensive. With this information I suspect correctly why he's slow, and seems mentally blunted. It's the medication load. He says to me, "I don't know if I can afford to make this trip with such a huge drug bill over and above everything else. Paying to go through the Panama Canal for even a little boat is skyrocketing!"

Jack's neurologist had been in practice about 15 years. The professors at the medical center where she trained no doubt received grants from drug firms who manufactured the medications she learned to use. In addition, everyone in medical centers and in community practice has understandably emphasized, "Always protect yourself from malpractice!" It is the need for sales and profit by pharmaceutical companies, however, that has gradually shaped how, when and what general physicians or specialists prescribe. As a result the quality of medical care had deteriorated accordingly.

The trouble is we're not dealing with soaps, waxes and cleaners, but rather medicines that are capable of adversely effecting people physically, mentally, and in terms of the very way they live. The sale of drugs is seen as an insidious ugly form of commercialization, or just "business," when there should be thoughtful consideration for what doctors may actually accomplish with all these recently available medications. Let's simplify by saying, "too much of anything, especially too expensive, is not better!"

Jack, a general practitioner by the way, was still practicing two days a week. He said his patients tolerated his slow deliberate mannerisms knowing his ability to think was intact! He obviously was seeking advice from a fellow sailor he accidentally came upon, who just happened to be an expert on the epilepsies. (What Jack hadn't discovered yet, I was the self proclaimed "Lord Blears, of this aspect of neurology.")

Jack, I said, "On July 1, 1997, at the 22nd International Congress on Epilepsy, Dublin, Ireland, I argued primidone, trade name, Mysoline, "used properly," is by far more useful than drugs such as Lamictal, Neurontin, and other drugs that have come along in recent years. All the newer medications are "expensive non-primary drugs," recommended as add-ons to established regimens. Presenting this information required "approval of referees from 16 countries." In other words, somebody else in the world must have been in agreement!

"How about taking my advice and phasing down the Neurontin?" "You can do it gradually while you slowly replace Neurontin with Mysoline?" To help make my point I referred to that "anthropologist who handled the epilepsy in Camaroon," the one whom I met in Dublin, Ireland at the 22nd international conference on epilepsy. Jack began laughing when I said, "Excepting here and now on this very boat dock, during 2002, only in Camaroon would you be getting such good advice." "How about it, Jack?"

Jack began phasing down his 1200mg. daily load of Neurontin. He wrote his own prescription for Mysoline and began cautiously with just 25mg. after his evening meal. About three weeks later, by chance, I bumped into Jack on shore. I didn't recognize him! He spoke out, was bouncy, acting very much the regular guy! He moved much more quickly, in fact seemed extremely lively and said in a clear quick voice, "I feel great, and quickly adjusted to Mysoline 125mg. twice daily. I'm still taking the other medicine, but I am off the Neurontin entirely!" "Any threats or odd feelings, or, anything that might be considered a warning of some kind of seizure symptom," I asked him? "None at all, and what a financial savings!" Jack said.

In all my years of private practice beginning forty years ago, I have never witnessed anything like Jack's transformation! Jack, fellow MD, seemed so happy he was ready to perform handsprings! In three weeks Jack had come from sounding and acting "retarded," from side effects of a combination of expensive medications to completely normal (!), and with a remarkably reduced drug bill. Now he seemed ready to sail for Panama, and oh, I was relieved?

It can take time for physicians and patients to get it right. A medical journal tells of the discovery of a blood platelet "sticky factor" called Thromboxane back in 1971. Subsequently Thromboxane is mentioned some 2000 times in the medical literature! However, it takes till 1977 for one of nature's own stroke preventatives to be identified and given a name, Prostacyclin. Prostacyclin is produced within the nucleated smooth muscle cells lining one's arteries. In normal lungs, for instance, there is what might be called a "protective Prostacyclin drip." Thromboxane, a clotting factor that opposes Prostacyclin, on the other hand, is carried by platelets that have no nuclei, and as a result are unable to produce it while they circulate. The platelets, however, can supply it for as long as they live in the circulation having a life span of three to 11 days.

Between 1972 and 1978 thousands of people allowed themselves to be misled and simply overdid it with Aspirin! Many suffered consequences like, for example, gastric bleeding. In fact, with too much Aspirin in one's system, unless neutralized (buffered), it was bound to interfere to some degree with the benefits of one's production of Prostacyclin! But how, until 1977, was anyone, anywhere, any place able to know that?

In the late nineteen seventies the "strategically most effective daily dosage of Aspirin," to combat the "sticky factor of platelets, to the extent of being a stroke preventative, was calculated to be 78mg. Commercially then "baby Aspirin" gradually came on the market at 80mg. A reasonable alternative was to take a regular size Aspirin, 324mg. Wednesdays and Sundays, or, twice a week.

In recent years drugs superior to Aspirin for preventing blood platelets sticking together or "clumping" during provocative circumstances, included Ticlid and more recently Plavix. Having never prescribed either drug, a patient familiar to me did very well on Ticlid for three years. He was then switched to Plavix without documented reason. Another patient, a pharmacist, treated with Ticlid experienced gastrointestinal side effects! Plavix has been a kinder drug for most people, better too probably, but considerably more expensive than Aspirin, and with a similar side effect profile as age old familiar Aspirin.

The strategy I learned and began in the late nineteen seventies, for prevention of little temporary strokes called transient (focal) cerebral ischemic attacks (TIAs), included Aspirin 324mg. twice a week, together with a nineteen fifties gout remedy taken daily, sulfinpyrazone (Anturane), said to toughen blood platelets, and dipyridamole (Persantine), a sixties coronary vasodilator medication that also inhibited blood platelet clumping.

During the eighties cardiologists, as a group, switched back to prescribing Aspirin alone. The collective opinion emphasized it was just as effective a TIA preventative as the three medications I used in the late nineteen seventies. If true, it was a money saver. By 1999, however, a supplement of the PDR 2000, featured a capsule known as Aggrenox, recommended twice daily as a TIA preventative. Aggrenox consisted of just 25 mg. Aspirin and 200mg. Persantine! The opinion of those who adopted to prescribe Aggrenox emphasized it was more effective than the daily 80mg Aspirin. By reducing the "aspirin component" to 25mg. consensus of current opinion indicated that Persantine was most important. Aggrenox, you guessed it, was expensive.

A 55year old acquaintance nearly died from a brain shower of tiny fatty particles from his heart, aortic arch or carotid regions. The event provoked platelet clumping, cerebral arterial constriction, and impaired circulation to his brain. After a stormy course, given Ticlid, he recovered remarkably well much to my amazement. Hearsay, he refused to give up smoking, although he may have cut down. Naturally friends and neighbors told him he's crazy not to quit entirely! His wife was beside herself but she also smoked, admitting he also really enjoyed a cigarette. This raised two imponderable questions, since smoking a cigarette meant so much to him, "Was it absolutely the best advice for him to entirely quit smoking? Was he smarter than his critics by choosing not to quit his "enjoyable habit of smoking cigarettes entirely?"

Smoking cigarettes points to nicotine. Nicotine, the oil as previously mentioned, is a deadly poison when absorbed through the skin. Nicotine is used in chemical warfare as a rapid paralyzing agent of nerve cell networks (ganglion blockade). There is no antidote for nicotine poisoning. Nicotine is also used as an insecticide. On the other hand, an "infinitesimal amount of nicotine in tobacco" is clearly beneficial for a number of reasons, according to millions of smokers of cigarettes. Rather than use up a precious water supply those who journey through the desert by caravan stimulate production of saliva by smoking a cigarette. Do you think you can persuade caravaners to stop smoking? Nicotine is one of the most fascinating molecular structures studied over the past 100 years! It needs to be considered separate from other ingredients in tobacco "smoke" that includes small amounts of carbon monoxide, nitric oxide and aromatic hydrocarbons and some other substances known to be able to incite cancer.

Nicotine is known since early in the 20th century to incite (delayed hypersensitivity more recently considered) one specific illness that usually comes on between ages 20 to 40 years and occurs in men 95% and women only 5%. It's Buergers' disease, or thromboangiitis obliterans, yet the nicotine effect spares one's coronary arteries (!), while circulation in limbs is gradually constricted. The "why" of this is open to much speculation. The "why" amputees, who suffered from Buergers' disease continue to smoke remains of psychological interest. Stemming from all this began a campaign against cigarette smoking in the nineteen twenties. Smoking cigarettes, however, is not thought of as "the underlying cause of Buergers' disease." An infinitesimal amount of nicotine inhaled in a cigarette, nevertheless, seems to directly cause peripheral arterial and venous inflammation as well as arterial construction in those who have this peculiar genetically programmed condition.

So, during the nineteen twenties, nicotine was recognized as a peripheral vasoconstrictor! As a result many physicians avoided the habit, but not all of them by any means. In the nineteen forties a carton of cigarettes made a nice Christmas gift for anyone, even some doctors. During World War II Camels and Lucky Strikes, along with coffee, helped soldiers motivate, suffer less hunger, think more clearly and remain calm, provided, of course those soldiers were accustomed to smoking.

After WW II toddlers were observed, in war torn Germany, trying to find discarded cigarette butts on the streets, or among the ruins, to return home and share a puff or two with their parents. Cigarettes were a major black market item along with first, "soap," followed by coffee and then gasoline.

In the nineteen fifties physicians analyzed the habits of smokers in terms of pack years. Two packs a day for five years equaled ten pack years. It was taught and thought by those at UCSF medical school anyone who smoked twenty pack years compromised his longevity without question! Emphysema and cancers of the lung were two main diseases that statistically related to smoking cigarettes. Lawyer Melvin Belli of San Francisco sued the tobacco companies! A warning had to be printed on each pack of cigarettes! Seymour Farber MD was professor of pulmonary diseases, and then head of that unit, for UCSF and Stanford at the San Francisco County Hospital. Tuberculosis, pneumoconiosis (inflammatory diseases, from breathing dust, associated with various occupations that led to fibrosis), and lung cancers were diagnosed, observed and treated. He said to our medical school class of 1958, "There may be a connection where smoking cigarettes and lung cancer is concerned but how do you explain the patients with lung cancer who never smoked at all?" He also asked, "Shouldn't lawyers have access to more information in order to be a little more "specific" before going to court with such an issue?" Unwittingly Seymour Farber was prophetic predicting the future of our US legal system as it stands today. Was a random petite jury of twelve, from various walks of life, supposed to provide "the final understanding regarding the matter of cigarettes and cancer and other chest disease problems?" A petite jury of 12 also agreed that "stress" caused various diseases, even cancer (!), so then, what if nobody in this very anxious world ever knew about tobacco and never smoked, would our life spans be, not longer, "shorter?" In the balance, has there been a positive side to smoking cigarettes that has been unfairly de-emphasized? How many people with huge waistlines became that way after they quit cigarettes? And, hasn't there been an increased statistical incidence of type II diabetes among those with gigantic waistlines?

Personally I never had an urge to smoke so it's a matter of watching from the sidelines. As the specialty of immunology has grown, diseases better understood, it has been verified that if too much is presented to the macrophages or "dust cells" that protect the lungs, they become overwhelmed, immune defenses start to cave in and serious disease(s) becomes the consequence. In other disease instances, the immune system overreacts and that may seriously harm or kill you unless drugs, that suppress the immune reaction, can be administered at that critical time.

As of 2002 nobody knows precisely what causes healthy cells to go wild, however, there are many clues. "Statistically" the medical literature is filled with speculative ideas as to what might incite cancer. One thing for certain, that medium sized star, or ball of gas in the sky known as our "Sun," our source on Earth of life giving (solar) energy, emits gamma rays that go right through us. Those gamma rays from nuclear energy challenge the DNA, within nuclei of the body's cells comprising some 100 kinds of tissues. This must challenge "transcription and translation of cells to stay on course." God knows! Cancer chemotherapy may have a success rate that can be likened to a good batting season for baseball however, when you think about it, it's amazing that it works at all. It does!

Does the alkaloid, nicotine, cause cancer? What about other alkaloids such as strychnine, quinine or morphine, do they cause cancer? Such questions are so vague as to be silly. Are the complete answers "yes" or "no?" Maybe watching television causes cancer. If our Earth is struck by a large enough object to jolt it off its' axis to put us closer to the sun, closer than the calculated perihelion of 91,377,000 miles, then maybe our worries about what causes cancer and who receives Nobel Prizes will be over.

Antibiotics are of great interest and also of immense value. Of interest three tetracyclines antibiotics are familiarly known as "chlor," "oxy," and just "tetracycline." They are used indiscriminately, and that's an understatement, and thus their effectiveness may be lost with resistant bacterial strains, and upon occasion, superimposed infections. Not depriving bacteria of their requirements, nor having the ability to destroy bacterial cell walls like penicillin, tetracyclines, inhibit protein synthesis. Of interest, for many years certain skin conditions are known to benefit from lengthy tetracycline programs. Is there anyone who hasn't at least heard about that?

As a favor, during 1999, I prescribed generic tetracycline, as a friendly gesture, to try to help a friend with a bothersome on going sinus drainage problem. I didn't prescribe methacycline nor doxycycline known to be more slowly excreted and, upon occasion, to cause "photosensitivity!" The patient, a nice lady, surprisingly, actually asked about photosensitivity as she planned to go somewhere to get some sunshine. Aware of certain patients given tetracycline for skin conditions, and also recommendations for those same patients, by dermatologists, they also get some sun (not a lot) for their skin condition (acne), I reassured the lady about photosensitivity. Based on the logic of what I knew from dermatologists, photosensitivity was not a real concern with just plain tetracycline.

Filling her prescription at Rite Aid, the pharmacist automatically included the drug warning printout. Of all things it warned, "May cause photosensitivity!" The lady, of course, called to notify me right away and naturally questioned what I had said to her. Instead of focusing suspicion on the validity of the printout, she naturally thought I gave her misinformation! Remember now this prescription was a "favor for a friend," and not a result of a paid visit. She even asked her sister, who reportedly commented, "Well, doctors don't know everything!" Not having denied that, since it's absolutely true, nonetheless this kind of a situation hurt my feelings as I think it would any physician. What has been programmed on a computer screen in the form of a drug warning printout was not open to discussion. It was not to be disputed. Physician experience, as rendered by the computer then, was meaningless?

With a "retired California physician's license," and therefore time on my hands, I dropped in on the Rite Aid store and with just a tinge of visible anger asked the pharmacist, "When did you start practicing medicine?" The pharmacist, somewhat shocked, his assistant also noting I'm upset listening to my grievance replied, "We are sorry, doctor, but we have no choice! The pharmaceutical firms absolutely require the warning printout with every prescription! It protects drug companies, and pharmacists, from (product liability) law suits." I asked both of them, "Have you every heard of photosensitivity from 'generic' tetracycline?" (Neither one could answer the question.) "Why the warning for "all" tetracyclines? They both reply, "We don't know doctor! Lawyers representing so many suit happy people?"

Thanks to the vicious and lengthy nature of so many malpractice actions and, understandably pharmaceutical companies and pharmacists desiring legal protection, same as doctors, it seems as though the devil himself frequently surfaces to show its ugly head. Even retired physicians tending to be generous with information, who offer the occasional prescription favor for nice people, need to be on guard and prepared, always, for the prospect of mostly senseless aggravation. It's best to know whomever you help well enough, and to be willing to keep a brief record of what you did, and why, just in case it ever becomes necessary to present what transpired in a brief charted form! That way, if you know what you were doing, you are going to be fully protected.

A pretty smart ophthalmologist, a sixties medical student from the University of Chicago medical school, tells me that his whole training experience probably took ten years off his life, even though he handled medical school, internship and residency, quite well. Exaggeration or not, four intense years of medical school is more trying than going to law school, a school of dentistry, pharmacy, or business school. Then, dealing with illness, you have many years ahead of you before you begin to "feel like you know what you are doing" and how important that is! Even prior to this day and age, with so very many drugs available (!) pharmacology, in particular, is a deficiency with every medical student. It's doubtful there are any exceptions. During medical school at UCSF I wrote only one prescription, and that was towards the end of my fourth year. During those four years I call "basic training," the emphasis was to learn to recognize the conditions, then you can dig in and "look up the treatment(s)."

As the practicing physician attends lectures to keep up, the hyping of certain prescription drugs leaves something to be desired. It's still the best policy for any physician to restrict the number of drugs he or she prescribes, and to carefully learn and remember details about each medication. The information is readily available. To instill confidence in patients, rather than doubt, it's important for a physician to know a great deal more about the medicine being prescribed, than to just know the medicine exists. Most patients, fortunately, detect you have this knowledge, and "acquire a therapeutic boost as a result." Most patients really appreciate it if it's conveyed you "know" something!

Not too many years ago it was a pleasure to practice medicine. The physician was given a good deal of respect, for knowing at least a few secrets of the human body, even as patients and their families faced nearly unbearable distress as well as untimely deaths. In the early nineteen eighties the confidential doctor-patient relationship became less respected. There was a growing emphasis on utilization of high tech machinery. Practice of medicine became even more compartmentalized. Too many specialists were routinely summoned to a hospitalized patient's bedside. Too many tests were routinely ordered. An ultrasound test to better define the problem, that may not have been serious after all, could have been ordered by the admitting physician if he knew enough and thought to order it. The cost of hospitalizations, not all necessary, increased steadily then went on to skyrocket, not just from over utilization but from stupidity. Mistrust among physicians increased, not just patients losing trust in their physicians, but physicians wondering just where they stood with each other! Perhaps three to five doctors saw a patient in a given hospital setting. None of them knew each other and, after seeing the same patient, never spoke with one another unless by accident. Each one, however, separately generated "hospital business!" Each one also could have written a prescription the whole scenario, supposed to be impressive, enough to scare anybody! Lots of tests with lots of opportunity to prescribe new and expensive medications!

On hospital wards pharmacists were placed on stand by. They were paid more than they deserved from insurance carriers, split with the hospital. The pharmacists became watchdogs for whatever physicians prescribed, to protect the hospital against malpractice suits. For office practice, the neighborhood pharmacist turned into the patient's advisor, especially since the patient was on medications from so many different sources. The pharmacist became increasingly relied upon, more understandable since the patient might be taking some medication his or her regular physician never heard of, and some medicines were outside the patient's regular physician's province.

By the nineteen nineties, adding more to physician misery, "Managed Care" called for a preposterous adjustment. The new setting narrowed the scope of thinking, and robbed physicians of enthusiasm for practicing medicine, defeating chances for improvement pertaining to judgment calls for better handling of patients. Medications, some physicians were accustomed to using in certain situations, were simply no longer available within the rigidly structured, cost conscious, managed plan.

Due to tremendous financial pressure, and obvious business investment reasoning by pharmaceutical corporations, the federal drug authority (FDA) tries its best to cope. Regardless, drugs are released for marketing that are expensive and no better than what's already available, except their hyped newness may have some psychological (placebo) impact. "With something new, then there's something exciting to do." Some newer medicines are for most even less desirable than medicines already available.

For the general practitioner unable to keep up, as well as a specialist using only medicines pertaining to one's restricted province, it might be macho but it's risky to be first in the community to prescribe a brand new medicine with just the knowledge the drug rep gave you. It's frankly amazing certain patients are so willing to try medicines with such lack of familiarity. In consultation some years ago, with a lady who came in carrying a bag with 17 accumulated medications, the pleasant lady offers no explanation whatsoever why she took any of her drugs, except several doctors she'd seen in the recent past recommended them! Checking her medicines it was a statistical miracle no conflicting drug actions were evident. Threatening to confiscate all of them, she didn't seem to mind giving them all up either.

For multiple sclerosis (MS) "gamma" interferon (IFN) has been shown detrimental. "Alpha" IFN was shown not to be useful for MS either. The third IFN, genetically engineered, has been touted as capable of preventing the flare-ups of patients with the most common presentation of MS, known as the relapsing-remitting form. In current use, has "beta" (IFN) been proven useful for relapsing-remitting multiple sclerosis, or, is it just considered safe enough to be hyped and offered to patients to take it in order to pay for the huge financial investment? Because of millions of dollars invested, products sold by salesmen and saleswomen, who have too little knowledge and no personal experience with what they are selling, are trapped in a frustrated new age where "hype" must be used to cope with a probability of unfulfilled expectations. Predicting when flare-ups of MS might occur is tantamount to predicting the future. Unless you have a very large group participating for years one may be fooled by statistics. On the other hand actuaries use past experience, and the law of averages to predict future outcomes, and that works!

Has tacrine hydrochloride (Cognex) really benefited patients with Alzheimer's disease, the disorder that has become a household word over the past 15 years? Cognex was first of three medicines that purport to make more acetylcholine (AcCh) available to improve memory loss. Only organic chemists or biochemists have ability for thoughts about this.

Acetylcholine (AcCh), constantly synthesized from acetic acid and choline, then instantly inactivated in the body, is absolutely essential biologically and chemically, for normal function of bowel, bladder, heart, eye muscles, skeletal muscles and the brain. There's no question about it! In fact, too much or too little acetylcholine paralyzes muscle functions, but, does a prolonged AcCh effect, targeting some brain receptors, help a patient to "remember" when, by definition, their normal brain tissue has already been transformed into abnormal sheets of aggregated fibrils called amyloid? It sounds like "snake oil." It really does.

Acetylcholine, along with other nerve transmitters within the normal brain is one chemical essential for "thinking," (Rat psychologist, David Krech, of UC Berkeley, showed this, in the early nineteen fifties, demonstrating clearly that his rats "thought" to run their mazes much better when "enriched with acetylcholine.") For "memory loss," however, to put it mildly, it's not very convincing to think that making a little more AcCh available, particularly at certain locations of brain receptors significantly changes anything. Another criticism, how many cases called Alzheimer's represent something else? Are brain biopsies being done to cinch this pathological diagnosis? Isn't it, nowadays, a diagnosis established by some "psychological test?" How does a patient with retarded depression do on such a test? Anti-depressants, like time tested Elavil, and of course so many newer drugs, are used in Alzheimer's disease rest homes. But how often do you discover someone attempting a therapeutic trial using triiodothyronine (Cytomel), l2.5micrograms to 25micrograms, to increase the benefit of a low dose of a tricyclic drug, like "inexpensive Elavil?" This approach, a late nineteen sixties prescription tactic introduced by psychiatrist, Morris Lipton, is forgotten probably because there is no longer any money in it! Cytomel, is still easily available but not as inexpensive as it should be because there's so relatively little call for it. Endocrinologists certainly must understand "the game." Other physicians don't because they are just victims of a modern commercialized teaching trend.

Cytomel or triiodothyronine (T3) governs one's metabolic rate, yet it's rarely used as compared to tetra-iodothyronine or levothyroxine (T4) that must breakdown into "T3" and T1. T1 must recycle back to one's thyroid gland in preparation for making more T4. Part of the reason some drugs are commonly prescribed like "Synthroid, Digoxin and Dilantin," it makes possible for laboratories to program and offer computerized sequential measurements of serum drug levels for certain popular medicines at an enormous profit!

The sales pitch directed to physicians to encourage ordering "drug levels" is that patients simply do not comply with medication recommendations. This is ridiculous based on my 35 years of office experience. Such profit, by the way, is not just for labs, but also for those who obtained "patent rights" for the technique. Physicians, with common sense, who know what they are doing don't need drug levels, unless of course a patient is unconscious, or unable to offer any information, with drug overdoses suspected, in which case the lab measurements become very valuable.

More careful, more thoughtful, and much less expensive ways for practicing medicine are for times gone by. Better medicine comes "without the hype for drug levels." Physicians relate much more closely with their patients under such circumstances. Even "Joe, the bartender," can tell if a familiar patron is on a third or fourth drink, and whether he or she should risk driving a car upon leaving the establishment. "Joe" neither requests nor needs any alcohol blood level! It's the "brain cell level of alcohol" that matters anyway, and that in part has to do with how quickly one's liver transforms the circulating alcohol into sugar (glucose). The societal problem goes on.

Before most physicians ever heard of a drug called Tamoxiphen (Nolvadex), "world class weight lifters and weight throwers" used it. They learned it was effective for treatment of gynecomastia (male breast enlargement). This undesirable side effect was associated with necessity for taking anabolic steroids, usually more than one kind (Testosterone, Anavar, Decadurabolin, etc:), in order to heavily weight train up to 30 hours per week! Without the anabolic medications such "genetically gifted athletes" were not able to advance further only able to train heavily ten hours per week on average. Ten hours per week weight programs proved hopeless to make necessary gains to qualify to enter even "trials" for world competition. No side effects from tamoxiphen were ever brought to my attention by these "full time jocks." Nolvadex seemed quite safe. The anabolic steroids were also apparently quite safe. In fact, anabolic steroids commonly used had an apparent wide margin of safety based on what I observed, in sharp contrast to other drugs, for good example a commonly prescribed drug for heart failure, digitalis. Digoxin, has a very narrow margin of safety. Many steroid athletes" overdosed themselves," before establishing their individualized most ideal "recipe," to enable them to train extensively with accelerated skeletal muscle recovery, and without apparent ill effects. This was in sharp contrast to digitalis, the most effective dosage very near the dosage that causes dangerous toxic side effects, i.e. "a very narrow safety margin."

During the nineteen nineties tamoxiphen became well known for treating estrogen receptor sensitive breast cancers. In other words it was shown useful combating glandular breast cancer when such tumor growth was judged to be very estrogen sensitive. Was it a great idea, though, to organize a trial for thousands of women to find out if tamoxiphen "prevented" breast cancer? Was it a good idea for those women who had a strong family history for breast cancer to enter in to that kind of trial? Common sense raised doubt, however, there was no doubt such a proposal supported the technology of mammography, and generated millions of business dollars.

Thousands of women, who were "not of identical genetic make-up," who by virtue of their mother having had breast cancer, were "convinced" they eventually would get breast cancer as well. In other words they were frightened into participating. They took tamoxiphen 20mg.daily, and after five anxious years on tamoxiphen (!) there was no preventing of large glandular breast tumors, or tumors of breast ducts. Instead, prevention of small tumors, growth sensitive by virtue of estrogen stimulation, was confirmed. That's why the drug was selected, and shown useful for the treatment of estrogen sensitive breast tumors, in the first place!

There were some side effects from the tamoxiphen trial. Taking tamoxiphen regularly for several years associated with a small, albeit significant, increase in uterine cancer. There was also an increase in vascular disease, from thrombosis, especially deep leg vein thrombosis. That was why women, considered prone to venous thrombosis, were dissuaded from participation in the tamoxiphen trial, instilling then, in such women, still more anxiety! Women, who didn't qualify for the trial, continued to "worry" even more about breast cancer, since they were denied the opportunity to take something to prevent it! It had to be emphasized to them what might happen if they took tamoxiphen. They were told of possible unexpected pulmonary embolism, with the threat of sudden death even if treated in time, because of an encouraged presence of deep leg vein thrombosis. Was the trial then worth it? What was the benefit except for "business," and in the course of creating such business what about creating so much anxiety?

A question was raised by the trials, "Does tamoxiphen "cause" uterine cancer?" No, it doesn't "cause it" but, by virtue of upsetting natures' balance, the incidence of uterine cancer, particularly in women with strong family histories of cancer in various tissues, appeared statistically greater compared to those who received a placebo or a sugar pill.No answer was available prior to breaking the double blind code of the trial, since neither physician nor patient knew who took the tamoxiphen, and who received the placebo.

What should a person worried about getting a disease do? It's a personal decision. To ask for an opinion about a proposed cancer preventative trial is rather like asking Alan Greenspan to help you decide if you should invest your savings in Procter and Gamble? As head of the Federal Reserve Board, that Board makes a decision to lower interest rate demands from the nation's member banks, but is that a guarantee your stock investment will grow? It certainly isn't!

Commercialism in medicine deserves a lot of criticism. The pharmaceutical industry seems to have reached a point of no financial consideration for consumers whatsoever! People are frightened to a point of needing a medicine! Millions of people are "attracted to drug products from television advertising." Because of the "power of television," the US Congress could do a big favor for the American public by passing a law that prevents "medicines" from being advertised via the television medium. If Congress passed such a law it would translate into a boost for "television supported by private donations." Imagine the savings, with so many TV advertising dollars no longer added on to the cost of drugs to consumers, as a result of passage of such a law!

Aren't physicians the ones who are educated for deciding which patients benefit from a medicine and who doesn't? Even if you think your doctor is "as dumb as an oyster," remember your doctor went to medical school, and you didn't! At least your physician knows the "language of drugs and medicine." You don't. Please, just give the whole matter a little more thought. Don't be bashful. Ask your doctor if he knows what he or she is doing! If this brings a laugh and the comment, "I hope so," you are on the right road to a good doctor-patient relationship. Of course doctors don't know everything!

It's not the local pharmacist, who labels and packages your medicine, making the big profit either. It's the CEOs and higher management, their lawyers, along with distributors of drug products, and pharmaceutical lobbyists that make up the list of profiteers. They don't know who consumers are so how could they know whether some consumer really "needs" the drug? It's just statistics, and you don't know if you "need" the drug either! You may know you "need something," and that's about it.

It's quite amazing how the non-steroid anti-inflammatory drugs (NSAIDs) relieve pain, via peripheral mechanisms, in contrast to morphine and opiate related pain relievers that work through the central nervous system. Morphine for pain, especially the horrible pain associated with terminal cancer, remains the most effective. Doctors should be alert, however, regarding "federal regulations!" But why should things be this way in view of so much suffering? "Give everybody an inch and they'll take a mile." Is that it?

Regardless of much deserved criticism, the future for medical care in order to improve is very much in the hands of the pharmaceutical industry. Cancer chemotherapy is disappointing because, like a batting average in baseball, it works its miracles perhaps only a third of the time. The fact, as aforementioned, such approaches work at all is amazing, and should boggle the mind at least a little. The skyrocketing cost of medical and surgical successes and failures also boggles the mind, and how!

There is no danger of newer medicines replacing the many indications for surgery. The appendectomy is not obviated because penicillin came along, but for awhile during the nineteen forties physicians thought it might be. Aseptic necrosis of one's hip, due to the ever so gradual diminishment of blood supply to the neck of the femur, particularly in alcoholics and persons who have had extensive anti inflammatory steroid therapy, is not likely to be prevented with medication any time soon. Strangely enough it is still not fully understood since 80% of the blood supply to the neck of the femur comes from within the femur (the bone) itself, a subtle ever so gradual and mysterious process, with bone turnover known to be about five years.

Expect great things but beware of the hype! What's disturbing for physicians is that it's gradually getting close to a "manufacturer to you drug delivery system." Many PhDs re-arrange atoms or radicals around molecular configurations (already shown to work), working, on computers for a "new design," regardless of how subtle, so that a "new patent" may be obtained along with great future profit, provided the "new designer drug" really works!

It's not surprising in spite of strict regulations, and substantial penalties, to hear of inside trading. Michael Douglas makes the point in his movie, "Wall Street?" The game of the rich is too get richer and it is "a game." They can't help it. It doesn't seem to matter that others persuaded to go along with the hype to manipulate stock value upwards lose their investments. The name Merrill Lynch seems to always pop up in scandals because they are the biggest among investment firms. One of the most publicized involves Imclone's drug named "Erbitux," promoted as an anti-cancer miracle. Perhaps the drug gets its name because "someone wearing a tuxedo stumbled onto a non-woody plant that produced a special herb." At any rate the FDA is not impressed. Newspaper articles nation wide report the CEO of Imclone "sold his shares profitably," learning right away of FDA's rejection, and Martha Stewart sold hers at a strategically profitable moment as well. Comedian Jay Leno reflexly incorporates such events into his mirthful material and Martha "has her tit caught in a ringer!" Well Martha is a very bright lady, but, she is not a physician and so my reaction is "What else is new, and why sadly would anyone invest in something as unlikely as Erbitux?" It shows how little they know. It's just betting.

What "is" disturbing is inside trading I suspect goes on involving medical center professors that possess advance information on a drug they will be testing. If early on there is some usefulness, the professor invests. Scientific editors of newspapers tout the drug. An expensive ad in newspaper classified sections at the very same time makes readers believe the product might be the "coming of a second penicillin!" The reader invests money and more and more is invested in conjunction with the hype. The university professor, however, sees only limited value of the new product and thus sells his or her investment at just the right time, to make a good profit at the expense of many others lured to believe the drug is a real break through. Here we have "conflict of interest," and the "intent to rake in money at the expense of innocent believers," especially within families hoping for help because someone of their family suffers the very condition for such medicine. One example is the drug selegiline ("Eldepryl") for Parkinsonism, a condition within my specialty of special interest.

In conjunction with one of my professors at UCSF, John Adams, Gugenheim professor of neurosurgery and chairman of the department, we shared an investigation number for the drug (IND) registered with Calbiochem and Eaton labs for l-dopa before the FDA released l-dopa in 1970. I gave the television show in Los Angeles sponsored by labor leader Joseph T. DeSilva (Retail Clerks Union 770) spurring FDA's release of l-dopa a mainstay for treating Parkinson's. John Adams was wonderfully inquisitive, a neurosurgeon and an intellectual, the son of a professor of philosophy at UC Berkeley. (Hopefully John is fine since retirement.)

To Michael J. Fox, "Thank you for your effort to raise research money for everyone with your condition! I have wracked my brain for years trying to figure out "why" we are unable to help cases like yours so much more. I apologize! It is simply beyond my brain's ability as "somewhat of an expert." If many "experts" got together and worried less about who gets credit maybe then comes your answer! Oh, by the way it's not Eldepryl. It's okay, but not the answer we are looking for!

Lastly, speaking of drugs that "do really work," and just when biologically oriented psychiatrists were convinced Sigmund Freud, distanced by Jung and Adler, was "down and out," along came Viagra! Who would have thought working with a cardiovascular CHNO configuration that reduces blood pressure via smooth muscle relaxation that caused erections as an unlikely side effect, could be rearranged into another CHNO configuration, that predictably led to an erection about 80% of the time (!)? (In fact it was the unexpected incidence of erections in old timers that held up FDA's release of l-dopa!)   The one proviso with Viagra you had to have "sex on your mind!" All that was additionally required was some kind of sexual stimulation. Well, Freud once said "sex" was on the mind of most folk 95% of the time! And even if Freud exaggerated (maybe it's only 91%), to make his analytical point, how else does one explain hospital educational seminars filling up! For impotence and Viagra it's standing room only, and following its release by the FDA radio and television talk shows burgeoned to such an extent it could have taken everyone's mind off Middle East oil? Hat's off to Sigmund!

As an alumnus of UCSF, a flyer comes in the mail about how things are progressing. Specifically it says, "The Genentech building on the Mission Bay site in San Francisco, 1 "DNA way," is bigger than the Salk Institute, in La Jolla, California!" What that really means, in terms of trickle down benefits, towards preventing and treating illness remains to be seen. How many "Salk equivalents" will be at work inside? Let's hope there is at least one. Let's be optimistic, and imagine there's ten! Jonas Salk, who I came to know personally, one day comments, "Had the 'legal system,' now in place, been in place in the nineteen fifties, there simply would not have been a Salk vaccine available to the public!" Such a vaccine, 100% effective, harmless to normal people, would be ruled "illegal! "Contracting paralytic polio, and living in an 'iron lung' would of course be 'legal'. " Is anyone in Congress thinking about changing the US legal system a little?   Is it possible there really "is" room for just a little bit more consideration and improvement?

It's a matter of intelligent "thinking," "correct motivation," "attitude," and "economic common sense." We can't increasingly skip on past what's really good for all us folk here on earth as improved technology encourages we focus our gaze at the Milky Way. If we get too caught up heading in that direction, there's a risk of becoming suddenly "unplugged," to discover we as a society are no longer able to even pay the utilities!" Then depleted of necessary funds we just slide ever so slowly backwards towards the dark ages, having to wait another few hundred years until again, there begins some future "age of enlightenment" with intelligent human beings hoping for another renaissance.

CHAPTER VII

"RITALIN, THE BRAIN AND VARIOUS 'STIMULATING' STORIES"

During the nineteen sixties there was a great effort to discourage use of Ritalin in the nations' schools. Alternative suggestions seemed to fall on deaf ears. Any reasoning from an academic point of view just led to more frustration. The effort to downplay the need for Ritalin proved a failure in spite of support from the US Congress. Congressman John E. Moss (D), Sacramento, and Congressman John Schmitz (R), Santa Ana, both from California and very concerned Ritalin was being used much too often, proved open to any alternative suggestions for accomplishing the main objective without using a direct acting stimulant. Granted Ritalin was quick to act and logically teachers were pleased to see a disruptive child become more attentive and less restless otherwise neither the hyperactive child nor the rest of the class would acquire the benefits from classroom exercises. School psychologists were very much in favor of Ritalin. Neither psychologists, nor those who measured student progress, nor teachers were concerned that Ritalin had become the most popular stimulant among pre-law and pre-medical students just before examinations.

In its favor, Ritalin is not physically addictive granted some professionals argue otherwise. In addition a good deal of the time it is effective for settling down the hyperactive student who pays little or no attention to classroom lessons.

Pediatricians proved always to be a closed group uninterested in listening to what other specialists had to say about medicines for children. No one except pediatricians knew about kids and if any opinion came from any physician other than a pediatrician it was not accepted. Psychologists specializing in children as well as teachers with no background whatsoever in pharmacology rallied around pediatricians. Even a sixties article in quite an excellent newspaper, the "Mercury" of San Jose, California failed to budge anyone. It mentioned prototype tricyclic drugs, imipramine (introduced by Geigy as Tofranil in 1959) and amitriptyline (introduced by Merck as Elavil in 1960). Working indirectly, absolutely non-habit forming, and given at home once daily, either or both used in children could accomplish the desired goal. Starting in very low dosages (10 mg. sizes) either drug that best suited the child was capable of transforming a disruptive youngster into an attentive one; the only catch is this indirect approach required a couple of weeks to take effect. The reaction to the article was that Tofranil and Elavil were "dangerous'" for children! Such an opinion was based on virtually no experience among pediatricians with either drug. Imipramine, marketed as Tofranil the anti depressant, was used very successfully for bedwetting (enuresis) by some neurologists as early as 1960. However, it took nearly 12 years for the pediatricians as well as many psychiatrists to catch on and discover it was apparently not "dangerous" for children or anyone else for that matter.

It remains important to remember one's central nervous system doesn't mature fully till about 16 years of age and thus Ritalin, for children, works its temporary stimulant benefit on immature nervous systems. In evaluating growing children the key word is "growing." some fast, some slow, some awkward, some outgoing, some reserved. Pediatricians invented the concept of "soft neurological signs." The word "soft" is attributed to schoolchildren diagnosed as having an attention deficit disorder (ADD). Describing ADD in this way proves more pleasing to concerned and disappointed parents. A youngster who in fact is "a disruptive jumping bean in human form," not revealing any "lateralizing signs" upon clinical neurological examination, is described as exhibiting "soft signs." For those ameliorating soft signs, Ritalin by 1999 is touted as "selectively able to energize a growing youngster's putamen!" the putamen a distinctive body within the central nervous system motor network. Logic says the action of any stimulant drug is hardly restricted to the putamen!

Without splitting hairs or pharmacological irrelevancies Ritalin is nothing more than a weak form of amphetamine(s) with a chemical designation methyl-phenidate. Like amphetamine Ritalin is a stimulant, albeit a weaker stimulant. In the countrywide sales race so far as I know Ritalin mostly replaces meth-amphetamine known better by its trade name Desoxyn. Sociologically, this is probably a good thing. Desoxyn is also known on the street as methadrine with slang names "meth," "speed," "crystal," "crank," and "white cross tablets." Another amphetamine derivative street drug, said mostly imported from Amsterdam Holland, is a drug that accelerates release of serotonin in central neurons known as 3,4 Methylenedioxymethamphetamine (MDMA) or "Ecstasy." Known since 1912, when it was first synthesized and finally used in the seventies in psychotherapy, Ecstasy is now increasingly used by youngsters who dance to music accompanied by strobe lights emulating the "rave scene" that began in England in 1988. Complications of "raving" with Ecstasy along with "tripping" on the alternative to Angel Dust known as Ketamine, along with the date rape drug gamma hydroxy butyric acid (GHB), are seen more and more in emergency rooms throughout the country with close to 100 deaths reported thus far.

Both Ritalin and Desoxyn were used for years for the same challenging problem of how to succeed in teaching very inattentive youngsters. In their favor it is important to "treat first and talk later!" Psychiatric and psychological researchers balk at this, however, these researchers have little or perhaps no actual hands-on experience dealing with hyperactive children and their parents.

To digress a little, the adage "treat first talk later," applies to psychiatric medicine in general whether it be for adults or children. This certainly applies to "monster children."

A child with "borderline personality disorder" who "acts out" (behaves inappropriately for unconscious reasons) can become so hyper and disruptive as to drive parents to divorce! Suicidal gesturing on the part of the disturbed child, for instance charging towards a glass door, wears severely on the parent, especially the one who stays home while the other gets some relief by going to work. Usually it is the mother who is relentlessly "the victim of daily 'target practice' from morning till night." Even when parents and their testy youngster get through all this the worry never ends. Typically it is the mother who continues to worry as her disturbed teen winds up on the street sharing complaints with "druggies," alcoholics and the homeless. One hears about a teen not uncommonly feeling a little better after snorting cocaine, another very predictable stimulant and a rapid acting one at that which, like amphetamines strong or weak, eventually results as a rule in depression upon discontinuation.

Since the youngster who is disturbed does not listen it is folly to think issues can be settled via persuasive talking and listening sessions. Accordingly it isn't practical to delay a trial on medication. Adding to the difficulties and making things more unbearable, bystanders think one or both parents are to blame, then one parent proceeds to blame the other, as the argument ensues whether the child's problem is learned or simply genetic. Relatives, friends and neighbors, even social workers, who can only imagine what goes on within the household of a disturbed child, their vantage stemming from a reasonably normal family setting, are critical. Lack of empathy and harsh criticism as a result can become cruel if not unbearable for the mother of the disturbed child.

As with all stimulants Ritalin is classifiable as an appetite suppressant. For growing youngsters, unless there's an obesity problem, it seems more thoughtful to try to avoid any "diet pill." In agreement that Ritalin may not be a major offender, pediatricians touting Ritalin tend to reject any notion Ritalin affects a growing youngster's appetite. They cite as an argument some Ritalin child who grew to a height of six feet four inches, ignoring thousands of children of much shorter stature who have taken and are taking Ritalin. Who knows how tall all might have been if indeed their appetite for nutrients had not been curbed, if it was curbed? Admittedly all discussion remains academic.

Since the sixties it's well established within pharmacological and psychiatric circles that habitual use of amphetamines eventually depletes adrenaline and some of its precursors in nerve cell storage areas in their extensions known as axons. Such depleted nerve cells may be referred to as "spent shells." A psychotic state indistinguishable clinically from schizophrenia may result. Giving Ritalin the benefit of not causing such a problem, can anyone say with confidence long term use doesn't leave the consumer, sooner or later down the line, with a desire for "stronger uppers?" Is there no risk that Ritalin can start a youngster on a path of eventually leading to becoming a spent shell syndrome or experiencing an organic schizophrenic psychosis?

As with all pharmacological approaches, the advantage of any drug needs to be weighed in the balance against immediate and conceivably delayed side effects. Ritalin is a very familiar medication to pediatricians, teachers and child psychologists and, as a "plus," Ritalin has been around not just for children, but also for the mildly depressed elderly for a very long time.

Considering newer drugs being developed within our computer age think about potential problems arising from visualizing and manipulating drug structures by rearranging radicals. A new and improved design of an amphetamine related drug (any drug) is touted before physicians have time to evaluate the previous drug recommended. How then does anybody make an intelligent decision whether the new product is better for the problem? In terms of instilling confidence it is much better to prescribe out of experience. Over decades of usage and familiarity, Ritalin then remains a very reasonable choice considering the "stimulant approach" for hyperactivity and attention deficits.

Where did the idea begin for prescribing a "stimulant" for an already jittery, seemingly nervous and restless youngster? In medical training at UCSF, I sat next to E. Denhoff, MD, as a visitor at UCSF. He first related a paradoxical experience in the nineteen fifties a similar such a case being then presented in our teaching auditorium. It was an example of "Denhoff's post-encephalitic child." What was demonstrated was the reverse of pharmacological expectations. This post-encephalitic child was calmed by stimulants and made hyperactive with barbiturate sedatives!

While Denhoffs' surprising discovery to this day proves unquestionably fascinating, medical histories, to the best of my knowledge, fail to suggest attention deficit hyperactive children are representative of post-encephalitic disease. While there's some basis for sake of pure academic discussion, it isn't practical or good common sense to tell parents their attention deficit child represents the aftermath of some "sub-clinical" case of encephalitis. It's as if you are making up something without evidence it occurred.

Sub-clinical disease is usually reserved for adulthood. Pediatricians, and pediatric neurologists, are very aware of the consequences of measles or mumps encephalitis. Para influenza viruses causing croup and inflamed bronchi, especially respiratory syncytial virus (RSV) occurring worldwide can be fatal for infant, toddler or youngster. Recovery confers only partial, temporary immunity. Recurrent infections are still very evident in children, again the sub clinical cases reserved for adulthood. (As an aside, the struggle to develop a "safe" effective RSV vaccine to prevent para influenza infections has been on going at NIH for some 47 years lest anyone thinks solving these problems is easy.)

Adding to the surprise that "a stimulant can calm" is indirectly illustrated by the fact that narcolepsy, age onset typically from ten to 20 years (Gelineau, 1890), was treated with some success with amphetamines beginning in the nineteen thirties. The first medical journal report of amphetamine abuse as a result of such treatment dates to 1938. Narcolepsy, "abrupt onset" (!) of rapid eye movement sleep (REM or "paradoxical" sleep) lasts usually 10 to 15 minutes, whereupon one awakens refreshed. While it may be prevented to some degree with amphetamines, barbiturates that do abolish REM sleep that typically follows within hours of normal onset slow wave sleep have no place therapeutically for narcolepsy.

Getting back to the hyperactive child calmed by stimulants such is really only half paradoxical. In other words a sedative hypnotic such as a barbiturate, instead of paradoxically making the attention deficit child more active, predictably sedates the child. Using that tactic, while assuredly beneficial for the rest of the class, it is not going to assist the restless inattentive student to get his or her lessons. Ritalin remains the established quick therapeutic answer in spite of an indirect approach with tricyclic antidepressants that takes two or three weeks to work. Experience shows fear of dangers using prototype drugs, imipamine and amitriptyline, in children is unjustifiable.

Imipramine or Tofranil proved a smash hit for the treatment of bedwetting (enuresis) by 1960 or about a year after the drug was introduced and marketed as an anti-depressant. Using the drug for many years, for children as well as adults, it was not until 1971, or 11 years after the drug was used by neurologists for enuresis, that this usefulness of imipramine appeared in the pediatric literature. Even following their journal article pediatricians continued to persuade, and persuade each other, tricyclic medications were dangerous for children. Perhaps failing to start with a low dosage of 10 mg. was part of their problem. Instead of therapeutic trials the idea to increase urinary bladder capacity and keep urinary sphincters tight during deep (slow wave) sleep, there occurred instead many unnecessary spankings, launderings and extensive urological work ups.

Granted treating children may well have its special tricks but a developing brain is still a brain whether neuro-chemical circuitry or interrelating biochemical compartments are fully mature or not. There are "excitatory" and "inhibitory" pathways and you may influence one or the other but you cannot influence both at once along the same circuitry. "Inhibiting inhibition" produces more excitation. "Exciting an excitatory pathway" produces greater excitation yet! If, on the other hand, you "excite inhibition" you induce more inhibition (calming)!

Rather than amphetamine related stimulants, imipramine and/or amitriptyline medications accomplish attentiveness and calming in less than a month with a much better future outcome compared to daily use of stimulants. An "amitriptyline child" is going to have a better wake-sleep cycle, logically be more refreshed, and therefore be apt to become a more attentive student than a Ritalin child. As a result the child adjusted to amitriptyline is more likely to proceed on to college than a "Ritalin child." This opinion of course is in accordance with my limited experience, all acquired indirectly as related by schoolteachers who feared Ritalin and instead accepted amitriptyline or imipramine, or a combination of both as an alternative for "their" children.

While it's fun to explain a little about neurological circuits, brain chemistry and pharmacology nobody knows how the brain works. Even tedious experiments that involve only vision shows that one eye is competing with the other eye thus there's "binocular rivalry." The "rivalry," however is neither within the eyes (the cameras) nor within the posterior part of the brain that "sees" (the visual cortex), but is instead somewhere between. The function of the brain may never be completely explained. If one day it is explained and in fabulous detail how then does one go on to explain the "mind?"

The human brain is "not" like any computer. The chemistry of nerve transmission is slow! Computers are fast. A "thinking mind" prefers, ignores, deliberates, forgets and of course remembers. The benefits from "forgetting" are immense and should not be underestimated. A computer is improved if it stores more information and presents the information faster. The brain (mind) flushes out unhappy thoughts and memories so that one's life in the future can improve. It's always possible with the human brain to achieve a happier outlook, make philosophical adjustments or perhaps even become enlightened, or, even go so far as to make a choice to get along better with neighbors, far and near, in this complex world. It's even possible to have no more wars; not likely, but "possible!"

Therapeutic discussions are helpful. Medications are often helpful. One adjusts and forgives or develops a new and different point of view. This may provide a more sensible, reasonable way to look at some situation. The human mind conceptualizes whereas computers are unable to achieve any intuited object of thought because computers do not think. Never mind singing the lyrics, "The best is yet to come and babe won't it be fine," because the best is already here provided it's used! It's your brain!

Evidence of the past half century corroborates the notion that the brain continues to improve if you exercise it as you would your biceps! With motivation to memorize one continues to acquire knowledge. The notion that the potential of the brain peaks in one's mid twenties is no longer considered true. The saying, "For every drink of hard liquor taken a brain cell dies," is not true. However you may give your liver cells too much to do and thus compromise your liver's ability to process the nutrients you eat in order to deliver those essential precursors to the brain or, for that matter, deliver essential factors derived from those nutrients to all your many organ systems. A faulty liver allows body systems to fail. From under-nutrition or the liver's limited ability to handle nutrients, depending of course upon individual differences, body systems like the heart, bone marrow, peripheral nerves or brain become compromised. Is there any reason "'boozeheimers' disease" couldn't cause, beyond the classic features of chronic alcoholism, "dementia with Alzheimer's-like changes," in the brain (plaques and neuro-fibrillary tangles) observed using 25 to 200 times the magnifying power of the electron microscope over the light microscope?

Considering how stimulants work, if Ritalin is not eventually a cause of a "spent shell syndrome," leading rarely to a schizophrenic like organic psychosis, are students who have been given Ritalin for years more likely to take stronger stimulants during street drug abuse later on? That is the big question. "If" true, then while Ritalin for say a year or two may help a young student obtain an education, it may set the stage for other problems that disable a person from using that education. It's a thought.

Can long term usage of Ritalin be a culprit that contributes to airway obstructive disease? Is there any relationship between a dramatic increase in cases of asthma in the younger population of the US and the prevalent use of Ritalin? If this is a thorny question it is nevertheless essential and reasonable to ask if you keep your pharmacological thinking fundamental. Recently at an educational conference for physicians in California an expert in allergic asthma dodges the issue, refuses to even speculate with an opinion. He replies, "I have no information on this whatsoever." Is the lecturer fearful of being criticized for offering an "opinion?" Can't "allergy" and "pharmacology" be mixed?

For any physician who wonders whether cocaine, the stimulant as used in the US, leads to airway obstructive illness it is now recognized it does! Several thousand young people die yearly from fatal asthmatic attacks. Crack cocaine, a very fast "upper" not only incites an asthmatic attack but is considered a "cause" of asthma! An explanation in part involves the immune system whereby four principle products of one's "lipo-oxygenase pathway" called "leukotrienes," that are able to severely constrict bronchial tubes, are released. Not only does constriction of bronchi occur but an increase in mucus secretions within the airway passages as well. Allergists consider this phenomenon similar to a "wheal and flare reaction" as seen in a positive skin test. Researchers in immunology focus on inter-leukins (biological response modifiers nick named "IL"s) "4" and "5" and "T-helper-2 lymphocytes" influenced by "smoked crack cocaine" to explain the underlying cause of the asthmatic attack.

The reason for drug abuse is the user wishes to modify his or her mental state. It makes sense that most abused drugs are those which exhibit a primary effect on one's central nervous system. Since drug abuse not only involves street drugs but also prescription drugs it is wise to consider, if possible, indirect rather than quick acting direct approaches to improve one's mental state and simply beg for a two to three week passage of time. In this way the treating physician steers patients clear of both physical and psychological addiction, the latter referring to "any habit that becomes a 'crutch' (smoking) that can be stopped provided there is a good enough reason.

If the chairman of the pediatric department (any department!) in any teaching center accepts a pharmaceutical grant (the same firm that produces Ritalin for example) isn't there going to be a tendency to tout that product? Isn't that the expectation of the pharmaceutical firm providing the money? How then does anyone in training in the department gracefully opt to try something different? Medical centers, now managed by banks to better collect and meet their huge payrolls, represent part of corporate America. Meeting rising costs and making a profit becomes the very essence of doing business. Why go into (any) business if you cannot make a profit? Should medicine be a business?

Currently the most recent Physicians' Desk Reference (PDR) is dated 2003 however it's the red covered new millennium edition for the year 2000, issued as "easier to read," that causes a chuckle. If within that "so much easier to read edition" the new pediatrician coming in to practice reads about "adverse reactions to Ritalin on page 2041" his or her inclination would be to never prescribe it! Pediatricians however are groupies. Benjamin Spock who lived a long interesting life is not around anymore. If you take a stand and try to be perpendicular you run too great a risk of soon becoming horizontal! If it's not social forces that do it, your wife will! Like most specialists nowadays, threatened by malpractice actions (meaning a lawyer locates then pays some willing physician to testify against you), more than ever it becomes a case of sticking with your group, accepting the vote (the committee usually meets monthly) and going along with the trend. It's called "keeping in step in your parade."

Lets imagine pediatricians now recognize the two prototype tricyclic drugs, imipramine and amitriptyline (traded for decades as Tofranil and Elavil) are preferred alternatives to Ritalin and make for a better approach over the long haul. Interestingly Geigy Pharmaceuticals that introduced imipramine in 1959 is now merged with Novartis pharmaceuticals .In the PDR Novartis provides information on Ritalin, but, displays only photographs of Tofranil-PM in sizes no smaller than 75mg., also in 100gm., 125mg.and 150mg.sizes! Without access to background information any pediatrician who prescribes "75mg." imipramine (Tofranil-PM) to start, logically assuming it must be the smallest size ever available, would likely run into big trouble both with his youngster and the parents! Where's the 10mg. Tofranil? Who makes it? It's not available any more? Then again, is it good "business" for Novartis to tip off a new pediatrician in practice about a drug available generically and quite cheap that might be better than Ritalin? Saving old PDRs isn't a bad idea. It gives one some perspective about commercialism and medicine.

If you read an older physician desk reference you wouldn't see that imipramine 10mg.in the morning with amitriptyline 10mg.in the evening might help some youngster acquire an efficient sleep pattern and thus the ability to be alert and ready to learn the lessons of the classroom, even amaze a teacher. Not too long ago, while shopping, a familiar schoolteacher waved to me and stopped to again reiterated how well her daughter did on Elavil 25mg.daily. Without the drug given to her daughter in the nineteen seventies, she felt sure she would not have completed high school. Instead she went on to finish four years of college and without any need for the medication!

More recently trained physicians, however, will sadly have been convinced and will emphasize to you that Elavil is an old drug (that's true) and while it was good in its day the newer drugs, they will say, are much better. This has been the effect of commercialism in medical centers where designer drugs and patents and the impact of money affect those training to become doctors.

An older drug is as good today as it was when it was released. Why wouldn't it be? Of course newer medications are going to prove to be better for certain people. Expensive drugs like Paxil, Zoloft and Celexa are going to be very effective for some, each one having selective features that will fit perfectly for a given patient. However, it's a good bet the 1960 drug Elavil begun in low dosage and raised as needed, will prove every bit as useful for a greater number of patients than all three of the newer medications aforementioned. "New and improved" may be valid for products used in your washing machine but not so with so many new pharmaceuticals since there is no way you can be so quick to judge "if your 'whites' actually got whiter."

The low dosage of a tricyclic drug didn't do the job in every case. During the nineteen seventies, the very time pediatricians, psychiatrists and sleep research physicians, particularly at Stanford, were touting "dangers of tricyclic drugs in children" a "monster toddler of a boy came to my office. He raised havoc in my waiting room during each visit consistently disrupting everyone! Finally 150mg.of Elavil brought him into the range of a normal toddler!   One hundred milligrams daily proved barely useful and smaller doses seemed of no value. It was clearly a case of Elavil, 50mg.three times daily or, "put the little guy in a cage and feed him through the bars!" Granted this was the only such case in 35 years of practice and it was unusual for such a large dose in such a small fellow to have not caused apparent side effects. Elavil 150mg.was a large dose for an adult, particularly when often times 25mg.for an adult served the purpose. The success of the case was a result of more than ten years experience with Elavil having used it not just for depression but as an adjunct for pain syndromes, as an adjunct specifically for migraine sufferers, and as a substitute for Ritalin, all with reported success from testimony of patients using various dosage levels.

Doses of medications rigidly set have equated with therapeutic failures and one must be careful even though it is rare that a low dosage of a medication can cause disaster in terms of side effects!   During the eighties, a case of ophthalmoplegic migraine (prior to her disabling headache, she was unable to move her eyes in a certain direction for perhaps 20 minutes) proved to be almost totally controlled with a combination of three medicines. This unusually cooperative lady in her sixties had read something about Lithium (not for mania but for migraine) in a lay publication, and for months urged me to add it to her drug regimen convinced the fourth drug would eliminate her headaches completely. To please her, because she was persuaded to believe that even Lithium alone would solve her headache problem, finally I went ahead and allowed her to add to her three medications "just one 300mg. Lithium carbonate per day." Two days later by luck I happened to be standing in my waiting room. The office was closed. She knocked at the front door. (A cottage near the Pacific Ocean) She aged 20 years within two days! She appeared at "deaths' door!" I said, "Sheila, what the hell have you done?" She replied, "Nothing, I've only taken one Lithium a day for just two days!" The Lithium was discontinued and within days she appeared again quite youthful for her age. (Presumably the Lithium interchange with intracellular sodium ion was responsible in part as there was no way to find out if Lithium in combination with her other three medications was somehow a significant factor.) Unbelievable!

Obtaining drug levels for "compliance" is just another form of commercialism and the tactic proves no match for seeing and talking at intervals with a patient you are treating. By requesting a "serum drug level measurement" to be obtained from a lab away from your office, should the patient be reluctant to tell the doctor having not followed directions, he or she restarts the medication after leaving your office. The drug measurement may not be obtained for a day, two or even three days after seeing the patient. It takes about three times the half-life of a medication to obtain a more beneficial steady state so exactly what is gained by getting repeated drug level measurements at labs away from your office? They may most assuredly not be reliable if the patient per chance isn't taking the medicine regularly as instructed. For the physician who is neurotic for obtaining serum drug levels he or she should randomly surprise the patient by obtaining a syringe of blood in the office doing the assay in the office or mailing it out to the appropriate lab. How often is the information obtained that way? Not often!

Completely unaware of politics I befriended two-time unshared Nobel Prize winner, Linus Pauling in the late nineteen sixties. The subject of nutrition had become his interest. The motivating factor for me was brushing elbows with someone who could teach me something. Linus, a very pleasant but forceful man, told me he entered the field of nutrition because there were many gaps in our knowledge of nutrients. Other fields of interest to him were already filled with excellent biochemists. Linus had already focused his interest upon so-called "megavitamin therapy" and emphasized that synthesized Vitamin C at $7.50 per kilogram was just as effective as pure rose hips Vitamin C at a cost of $1500. per kilogram! He had written a book about Vitamin C and the common cold that engaged a good deal of public interest, also criticized the medical profession.

Linus Pauling began taking three grams of vitamin C daily when he was in his mid sixties. Soon after, to prove a point vitamin C was safe to take, a Stanford medical student was paid to take a fifth of a pound of Vitamin C daily to demonstrate it was harmless. The student after two or three months reportedly experienced no ill effects and therefore registered no complaints. In fact he was happy to make the easy money.

Interning in 1958 I met Albert von Szent Gyorgyi when he visited UCLA Harbor General Hospital in Torrance, California to lecture on actin and myosin and muscle biochemistry. It was announced as part of our introduction that "Albert" discovered Vitamin C (in the adrenal glands) and for that, as well as other original work involving biological oxidation, he was awarded the Nobel Prize in physiology (medicine) in 1937. Gyorgyii, a most colorful man and certainly not lacking a sense of humor, was happy to shake "my" hand since I fitted in so well with his lecture being a regional champion Olympic games styled weight lifter. I won the Helms Award as best lifter in Southern California taking first place in ten consecutive meets measured as total poundage for press, snatch, and clean and jerk 198 lb.class. This was during the latter part of internship in spring 1959, with heavy training six hours a week, mostly Harbor General cafeteria food, no vitamins (no steroids) and not getting much sleep. (I could also run a 100yard dash in

10.5 seconds in regular footwear; not fast for an AAU track meet but fast for an intern and faster than any nurse! Professor Gyorgyi was impressed with my modesty.

In jovial conversation years later with Linus Pauling, appreciative of a laugh, he said biochemist Albert Gyorgyi assured him Vitamin C was "extremely safe in very large amounts, totally unable to understand why the medical profession determined it was dangerous." Linus got a kick learning I had personally met the "very man who discovered Vitamin C," especially with such a perfect opportunity for letting Albert von Gyorgyi know, while he was most assuredly smarter, I was definitely stronger and had "more actin and myosin, 'at least peripherally'!" (Unless you are a biochemist you would not be apt to laugh at that statement. It really is quite funny.)

As a result I began three grams of Vitamin C daily along with Pauling and have taken that daily dosage for over thirty years, without regrets, as a salute to Albert von Szent Gyorgyi and Linus Pauling whether "in 'need' of that much" or benefiting from such a mega dose or not. It doesn't matter! It was well established that 3000 mg. of daily Vitamin C constituted 2,970 mg. over the established minimum daily requirement (MDR)! Linus Pauling, by the way, eventually upped his to ten grams daily. (Vit. C powder: half ascorbic acid, half sodium ascorbate), then years later he had increased to 18 grams a day where I stayed with just three grams. (Everything in "moderation.")

On teaching rounds at UC Davis Sacramento medical center I casually mentioned I was regularly taking three grams of Vitamin C every morning. The interns and residents reacted with a startle. When doctors of the Sacramento Society for Medical Improvement together with the California Medical Association (CMA) heard I was taking three grams of Vitamin C daily they canceled my CMA radio show out of Sacramento! In addition to the rather dull CMA format about what to do for bee stings and haemorrhoids I had written seven more entertaining scripts, all approved except the one about Vitamin C. When I showed the Vitamin C script to the executives of the medical society, before airing the show, that did it! Without notification to me one Bill Duke at the radio station was requested to just lock the door to my space so I'd get the point! On top of that, as an attending clinical instructor of neurology at UC Davis Medical Center and one who actually helped form the new department, I was not renewed as part of the attending neurology teaching staff when my yearly appointment came up for renewal.

Why organized medicine was so fearful of any physician taking extra Vitamin C seemed weird and why for that matter wasn't I "allowed" to be friends with Nobel Prize biochemist Pauling anyway? Wasn't I permitted to be friends with him?

I telephoned Linus Pauling to let him know I was enthusiastically in the process of arranging a trial of three grams daily Vitamin C with the Teamster's Union! Such a human trial was to settle this issue (hopefully) once and for all by providing statistics on a very large scale as evidence that an extra daily amount of Vitamin C either has value or it doesn't. Linus commented, "there's no shame attached to any experiment that leads to a negative outcome if that ultimately does prove to be the case." Linus was very curious and naturally interested in learning what hundreds of thousands of Teamsters might report in their medical records after two years on three grams of Vitamin C daily and Linus did predict benefits, particularly in ameliorating the common cold.

Vitamin C tablets were to be made available at all truck stops for 1.4 million Teamsters. The Vitamin C trial proposed was for a minimum of two years. Its scope would hopefully settle the issue by determining through Teamster medical records (already established as quite adequate) if extra amounts of Vitamin C proved of preventative value for the common cold, for healing of injuries, or, seemed significant for whatever else speculated. Pauling was delighted! All the truck drivers interviewed enthusiastically agreed to cooperate. The "hitch," however, was that Jimmy Hoffa had to give the okay and say, "Drivers, "Go ahead, pay for the vitamins, adding just a few cents to the cost of your meals. Let's participate!"

I had a very upbeat telephone conversation with the prison warden at Lewisburg penitentiary in Pennsylvania who said he enjoyed our talk very much assuring me he would relate my proposal on behalf of Linus Pauling to "Mr. Hoffa." In addition I got in touch with William Loeb in New Hampshire, (We became pen pals for ten years until Bill Loeb of Prides Crossing, Editor and owner of the Manchester Union Leader in New Hampshire passed away September, 1981.) William Loeb was a very close friend of Jim Hoffa. In addition I also became friendly with Sacramento's George Mock, an international vice president of the Teamsters, and occasionally his lunch pal at Machiavelli's. (Charlie Nichols and Bud Bryant of the Califronia carpenter's union often joined in to make the occasions simply fascinating for me and more stimulating by far than having lunch with doctors at Sutter General or Mercy General hospital.) I was very impressed by the seriousness of these union leaders. They were real leaders!

A two hour conversation with an investigative reporter of the Chicago Sun Times who had followed Jimmy Hoffa's trials and tribulations from the very beginning assured me Hoffa was "railroaded for political reasons." Hoffa was guilty, yes, but "guilty only of 'doing too much for his' truck drivers!" Expectedly, except to those within the Union that had tried every approach reasonable, Jimmy Hoffa was going to be released hopefully by the summer of 1971 following his scheduled federal parole board hearing. Hoffa's son, (now head of the Teamster's Union as of 2001), represented his dad simply because others had tried every angle and failed to obtain his father's release. During the summer of 1971 the federal parole board consisted of five members.

The five members of the federal parole board at Hoffa's parole hearing were: William T Woodward Jr., William E. Amos, Paula Tennant, Curtis Crawford and Maurice Figler who replaced Walt Dunbar in February, 1971. According to my friend John Hyland of Sacramento, former US attorney when Pat Brown was governor of California, Paula Tennant voted for Jimmy Hoffa being released from the Lewisburg penetentiary as did one other member of the federal parole board. However two votes for his release were not enough. Three voted against Hoffa's son's pleading for his father's release. It was obvious there was "political influence." In view of all the circumstances that led up to this summer '71 federal parole board hearing it was obvious those who voted against Hoffa's release reacted subjectively, not objectively. More accurately, it seemed some kind of collective judgment was made out of spite.

The vote not to release Hoffa at this critical time was totally lacking in foresight and also irresponsible "sociologically." It reminded one of the emotionality of some divorce proceedings where the woman wants to get the best of the man no matter if it is in her interest or not. By not releasing Hoffa at this critical time it was as if the federal parole board desired to punish every

Teamster because Teamsters liked Jimmy Hoffa! It put at risk the viability of the "Teamster pension fund." Everybody interested knew there had been "Teamster investments in Nevada operations." Wasn't it a very well established fact that there were hundreds of thousands of people who visited and "invested" in Las Vegas when breakfast cost a quarter and dinner about a dollar; a social system whereby a regular working stiff could feel like "somebody" for a few days? Does anyone who cares about the "little people" (people who "work" for a living) think Las Vegas is better now?

It was well publicized by 1971 that Howard Hughes had moved his operation to Las Vegas at the Desert Inn with primary interest in aviation focused on the Las Vegas airport. There were already established collaterally the "Hughes joints" that reflected, not unexpectedly, very different accounting procedures than other casinos established in Las Vegas over previous years. What was beneficial for expansion of the city of Las Vegas using the "previous accounting system" or the "new" proved of little importance to the FBI and the Justice Department who brought in the IRS to fight the Mafia to what Senator Paul Lexalt of Nevada called a "Mexican standstill." (How is it possible to trace "cash" anyway?) The short of it, had Hoffa been released, much of the mess of the nineteen seventies that involved bloodshed, as well as killings could have been avoided along with substantial preservation of the "Teamster's pension fund." A curiosity too was exactly why Walt Dunbar was considered unable to remain on the federal parole board through the summer of 1971. He, like Paula Tennant who reportedly voted for Jimmy Hoffa's release, was also from California. (Why wouldn't this at least raise some curiosity?)

The Vitamin C trial with the Teamster's Union thus never came about after laying all that groundwork! The results of such a trial involving vitamin C, though not "double blind" but "single blind" still, by virtue of so many participants, was estimated as having great practical value and certainly would have confirmed the safety of large dosages of Vitamin C. Organized medicine's adoptive viewpoint at the time was that even so much as three grams or 3000mg. Vitamin C daily was potentially harmful, everything from impairing Vitamin B12 absorption in one's stomach to causing the formation of certain kinds of kidney stones and other bunk. As for impairing Vitamin B12 absorption the notion simply proved eventually erroneous with the absence of molecular oxygen in the stomach not considered in their argument. As for kidney stones it was of interest many urologists had recommended ten grams daily of Vitamin C (ascorbic acid) to therapeutically acidify the urine. For such a therapeutic measure to cause a kind of kidney stone would have been a rarity indeed.

As for mega vitamin therapy the basic question simply was whether extra amounts of certain vitamins like E, C, B3 and B6 have value in certain people in a population sample. Some were convinced, based on anecdotal evidence, that extra B6 was useful for autism. The Shutes in Canada originally espoused, and later fitness phenomenon Jack La Lanne believed (still believes), extra lipid soluble Vitamin E was very beneficial for increasing cardiac endurance. Vitamin C, soluble in water, has received so much notariety it need not be elaborated upon. There were reports that extra amounts of Niacin or Niacin amide up to 30 grams per day (!) were upon clinical observation beneficial for schizophrenia. In some cases Niacin was used alone but most often it was Niacin in combination with mega doses of Vitamin C that "clearly seemed of benefit for schizophrenia," an opposing argument schizophrenics at times remitted spontaneously thus making the vitamin therapy coincidental.

To this day there are professionals dealing with mental illness who say mega vitamin prescriptions of three grams each of Niacin or Niacin amide and three grams of Vitamin C are without any value whatsoever implying the whole idea as being silly. This has especially been the case stated by those with absolutely no personal experience in this area of any kind whatsoever. One wonders how such people develop such firm opinions?

Out of respect for those in medicine proposing a mega vitamin approach to mental disturbances of all kinds, and in time convinced no harm could come of it, some 200 patients, adults but mostly children, were prescribed three grams daily of niacin amide along with three grams of Vitamin C. Anecdotal experience revealed striking behavioral improvement within days in, unfortunately, only 40 of the 200 patient trials. This 20% positive result, however, was based on the parents of children and their teachers in addition to office observations and discussion with the patient who took the extra amounts of the vitamins. What was a physician supposed to do, tell the patient he doesn't feel better when the patient says he or she does? For adults it was either a spouse or a close relative that noticed the dramatic improvement. Psychoanalysts again have been critical. They have claimed spontaneous remissions occur in 25% of cases of schizophrenia making any and all mega vitamin therapy benefits coincidental. Regardless, such improvement in the 40 cases cited, including cases of schizophrenia, timed with using mega vitamins B3 and C, provided a strong suggestion that this be tried in all cases of mental illness including schizophrenia, and as well in cases of attention deficit disorders and even personality disorders. Why not simply try it? Is there, especially nowadays, any legitimate reason for not simply trying this very inexpensive approach just to see what happens? And, by the way, I have personally respected the opinions of the Shutes in Canada and Jack La Lanne years before cardiologists themselves became convinced there was some cardiac value for taking more than the MDR of Vitamin E and have taken each day 400mg.for 25 years. I began when cardiologists called it vitamin Eeek!

New drugs emerging on the scene the last one to 20 years beginning for instance with Prozac and then Zoloft and Paxil (and others) selectively tend to target mostly serotonin, indirectly making more serotonin available for certain pathways. Of course they all have value for depression in a number of patients. The wonder drug breakthrough among prototypes of the tricyclic class of drugs, namely Tofranil and Elavil, stemming from fifties research, also promote serotonin and, in addition, nor-adrenaline to be available at certain nerve pathways. Elavil by gently reducing nerve re uptake emphasizes the serotonin pathways. If depressed patients in some third world country had just one anti- depressant drug (they simply couldn't afford to purchase the newer drugs anyway!) Elavil, the "gold standard," would be the wisest choice because, if used correctly, starting with 10 mg., Elavil is the most likely to help 50% or more such cases. Side effects are avoidable when the doctor begins with the lowest possible dosage and gradually adjusts the amount needed. One caution with Elavil where food is plentiful, is that it stimulates the appetite, the very opposite of fluoxetine or Prozac which is an appetite suppressant that actually relates pharmacologically to fenfenfluramine. Tofranil, at least in my experience, tends not to lean one way or the other in respect to appetite.

It's important to understand that nerve cells have re-uptake pumps and the six or so tricyclic drugs that reportedly solve about 70% of the depression problems of the elderly work in a way to slightly slow these "pumps." At the nerve ending, when an assigned chemical is being delivered to the next nerve network, the discharging nerve normally pumps back 80% in 7/100s of a second! If the tricyclic drug slows the re-uptake pump and then the cell takes back 79% or one percent less, then one percent more logically becomes immediately available. There is no depletion of stores and thus the involved nerve still remains able to maintain the essential chemical stores made from amino acids from protein in one's diet. This explanation gives the concept for a patient to think about.

Amphetamines are only minimally able to affect the nerve cell re-uptake pumps and essentially stimulate nerve chemical release. This is in contrast to cocaine that dramatically slows or even momentarily paralyzes re-uptake pumps likely flooding certain nerve pathways with adrenaline related nervous system chemicals! This is why cocaine, actually a very predictable drug, can be dangerous. A "thoughtful street drug pusher" (if you are willing to believe there is such a thing) makes a point with his "clients" to be very cautious and every so many years to plan on a cocaine holiday. In all fairness chewing a coca leaf like they do in Peru is hardly harmful, whereas smoking crack cocaine as so many do in America is quite risky.

To this day I've had a chuckle remembering the Merck-Sharp & Dohme pharmaceutical representative approaching during my first year of neurological residency at UCSF. He looked almost too serious as he explained Elavil as being a "very good product." Now 43 years later it has remained a very good product and, if used properly, a product apt to still help more people (for instance regulating one's wake – sleep cycle) than any other drug marketed for a similar purpose. Yet many physicians have regarded Elavil today as a medication that was simply good many years ago or in its day and a drug that has now been replaced by the newer and improved anti depressants. For the sake of making money, Elavil certainly has been replaced by newer patented drugs. To the physician with experience treating patients, particularly with a fiduciary responsibility, Elavil has remained the "gold standard."

For all in research, not only 'post docs' or Ph.D.s, but physicians who never practiced in the "trench," it seems more appropriate to "ask rather than give advice" on how tactically to win the battle of helping a patient in trouble. The three years old male toddler seemingly normalized on 150mg. Elavil is a case in point albeit a rare case. Elavil wisely used supports the notion of "treat first, talk (to the parents) later." Beginning patients on a very low dosage means you won't miss the "low dose responders." At the same time raising the dosage gradually and sticking with it, while observing that clinically unwanted side effects are not preventing you from doing so, means you will make the most of any pharmaceutical product.

Where children are concerned of course pediatricians are the experts. Why wouldn't they be? Children are their specialty. On the other hand is there really a good basis to prevent specialists from relating with one another? Why is it necessary for a neurologist or endocrinologist or psychiatrist to become a pediatrician in order to relate with a pediatrician? Is there some fear about sharing knowledge and experience openly?

At UCSF from 1960 to 1963 our neurology service was on the seventh floor of Moffitt Hospital.

The pediatricians were on the sixth floor just below and yet we never spoke to each other, and rarely were we put together for any conference. Has that policy changed over the years because there just might be some room for improvement.

ABOUT THE AUTHOR

Perhaps it is important for the reader to know this effort was written by a one time child of San Francisco who had no conscious thought of becoming a physician until 22 years of age and who considered it miraculous to be accepted to UCSF medical school in 1954. Being very distracted with many (other) interests it was puzzling, even sad, to learn of other applicants with better and some with nearly straight A grades who were not picked for one of the medical school's 76 seats. Among 1100 or more applicants, I wondered and still reflect on "why me?"

Unbeknownst to anyone at UCSF, except Dean Francis Scott Smyth, it was simply awful losing my mother five years later, when I was just eight years old, during April 1939. "The operation was a success but the patient died." She died of kidney failure (uremia) within 90 days." Physicians those years helped my mother the best they knew how as sulfonamides, available in Germany, were not available in the U.S. till a number of months after she passed away. The recommended therapy was to remove what was thought the most diseased kidney. However, there was no way at that time to determine which kidney was most diseased. Unfortunately she needed the best of both kidneys to survive and their ultimate strategy proved not correct.

Other writings include Weightlifting in Motivation in Play, Games and Sports, 1967, "Watch it, I might be dangerous" (49 people who made a difference), 1970, Cyrano de Bergerac, One Man Show, 1988, a number of published medical abstracts and letters on multiple sclerosis, epilepsy, one on drug induced malignant temperature elevation between 1977 and 1997.

1931	Born January 6, San Francisco, CA
1945	Bellarmine College Prep, San Jose, CA
1946	Lowell High School, San Francisco, CA
1947	Pillsbury Military Academy, Owatonna, Minnesota
1948	Turned down West Point appointment by Iowa Senator. Enlisted "Army" Air Force-Army basic training then Radio school.
1949	Radio Squadron, Darmstadt, Germany with cryptographic top secret clearance. University of Maryland Extension, Frankfurt.
1952	Entered U.C. Berkeley as sophomore speech major.
1953	KPIX, Ch. 5 commercials and leads in plays at U.C. Berkeley. Turning point: was five year contract offer as a television pitchman and another offer as news anchor, and television dramatic shows in Los Angeles. However, Duncan Holbert M.D., a paralytic polio victim stricken in his third year of general practice and living in an iron lung in Santa Cruz told me that I should be a "Physician"! He was such an inspiration, I agreed and returned to UC Berkeley immediately changing major to "pre-med" to show him I could do it.
1954	Professor of pediatrics William Reilly of UCSF invited me to his home one Saturday morning and told me during our visit with a chuckle I was accepted to UCSF as "Dean's choice" in 1954. I remember Dean Smyth interviewing me almost insisting I move out of the fraternity house and buckle down and if I could just get through the four years of medical school "without punching one of his professors on the nose," I would be a very good doctor. I thought then there must be feelings that all doctors are not necessarily good doctors.

1958   Medical degree UCSF.
1959   Finished one year internship at UCLA Harbor General Hospital, Los Angeles.
1960   Finished one year internal medicine residency at UCLA Harbor General.
1963   Finished three years neurological residency at UCSF, chief resident Fall 1962.
1966   Finished three years as the first neurologist in Newport Beach, CA.
1967   Finished ten years practice in Sacramento, CA. In 1966 I was the second neurologist to practice in that community.
1998   Retired after 35 years solo practice, the last 22 years in Laguna Beach, CA.
2001   Won U.S. national championship for Olympic style weightlifting for 90 kg. Class, age 70 to 74 (had previously won Helm's award in 1959 as best weight lifter in southern CA., 90 kg. Class. Also in 1959 won first place in all ten meets entered while interning at Harbor General on not so much sleep, no steroids and mostly hospital food.

LaVergne, TN USA
15 December 2009

167038LV00001B/36/A

9 780977 454112